Plant-Based Diet Meal Plan

Better Health and Energy in just 10 Days

Carl Jepson

Copyright © 2018

All rights reserved.

Table of Contents

Part 1

Introduction 1

Chapter One: What is Plant-Based Eating? How Does It Differ From Veganism? What are The Health Benefits of Eating Plant-Based Food? 3

Chapter Two: Clinical Studies: Science-Backed Proof 7

Chapter Three: Basic Four-Week Meal Plan 12

Conclusion 143

Part 2

Chapter 1: Obesity and the Standard American Diet

Chapter 2: Knowledge About Proper Nutrition

Chapter 3: Lack of Exercise

Chapter 4: Downfall of Medication

Chapter 5: Case Studies of Places with the Highest Longevity

Chapter 6: Who This Book Is For

Chapter 7: Leaky Gut Syndrome

Chapter 8: The Plant-Based Miracle Diet

Chapter 9: Benefits of the Plant-Based Miracle Diet

Chapter 10: Other Options and Diet

Chapter 11: Myths and Dangers

Chapter 12: The Importance of Nutrition
Chapter 13: Safety, Side Effects, and Warnings
Chapter 14: The Light Dieters

Chapter 15: Intermediate Dieters

Chapter 16: Hard-Core Dieters

Chapter 17: Going Organic

Chapter 18: Complement to a Healthier You

Conclusion

© Copyright 2018 by Carl Jepson - All rights reserved.

The following Book is reproduced below with the goal of providing information that is as accurate and reliable as possible. Regardless, purchasing this Book can be seen as consent to the fact that both the publisher and the author of this book are in no way experts on the topics discussed within and that any recommendations or suggestions that are made herein are for entertainment purposes only. Professionals should be consulted as needed prior to undertaking any of the action endorsed herein.

This declaration is deemed fair and valid by both the American Bar Association and the Committee of Publishers Association and is legally binding throughout the United States.

Furthermore, the transmission, duplication or reproduction of any of the following work including specific information will be considered an illegal act irrespective of if it is done electronically or in print. This extends to creating a secondary or tertiary copy of the work or a recorded copy and is only allowed with express written consent from the Publisher. All additional right reserved.

The information in the following pages is broadly considered to be a truthful and accurate account of facts and as such any inattention, use or misuse of the information in question by the reader will render any resulting actions solely under their purview. There are no scenarios in which the publisher or the original author of this work can be in any fashion deemed liable for any hardship or damages that may befall them after undertaking information described herein.

Additionally, the information in the following pages is intended only for informational purposes and should thus be thought of as universal. As befitting its nature, it is presented without assurance regarding its prolonged validity or interim quality. Trademarks that are mentioned are done without written consent and can in no way be considered an endorsement from the trademark holder.

Introduction

Every vitamin and nutrient humans need can be found in a plant-based diet… including B12 and protein… Yes, protein. There are countless clinical studies that show a person does not need meat or even cheese in our diet. Not only will your body thank you, but Mother Earth would be appreciative if it could be personified.

One-third of all freshwater is used for livestock, and almost one-third of ice-free land on earth is used to grow grains and produce that is not used to feed human beings directly. This is a large amount of resources going to livestock which is used to feed the Earth's inhabitants. In this book, you will learn about plant-based eating, how it differs from veganism, and how plant-based eating can change your health for the better. This book will also touch base on a few scientific studies backing the decision to go animal-free… as well as an explanation of vitamin B12, vitamin D, iron, and protein.

The consumption of dairy, eggs, and meat can cause a myriad of health problems, and you will learn how you can get all your daily nutrition without eating a typical American diet. Included will also be a 30-day meal plan just in case you were not sure where to start. Eating a plant-based diet was considered radical many years ago, and even though you are amongst a select few who choose plants over meat…your numbers are growing and hopefully will continue.

Chapter One:

What is Plant-Based Eating? How Does It Differ From Veganism? What are The Health Benefits of Eating Plant-Based Food?

When people hear the words, "plant-based eating," they usually assume they would need to sacrifice good food for healthy living… this is not the case. Not only do you feel great when you make the switch, but you will find the food to be delicious and quite filling. Being plant-based is not about just eating salad. Salad will be very boring… probably after the second one. There is not a single person on earth who will like salad that much. There are so many different varieties of foods to eat, you just need to be creative, and sort of learn how to cook. So, what is a plant-based diet, you ask? This is a diet that consists of the consumption of whole grains, fruits, vegetables, nuts, legumes, and beans. You will eat a lot of different varieties of rice and potatoes if you are not concerned about carb-intake.

Which brings me to discuss the difference between veganism and a plant-based diet: Veganism is defined as the rejection of all animal products and animal by-products to further prevent the exploitation and suffering of animals. It is a lifestyle that is not just a diet, it includes the rejection of clothing, shoe, household product, and make-up companies that profit or participate in the maltreatment of animal. The products they purchase are frequently stamped with an encircled "V" with the sub-title "cruelty-free" underneath it. This differs greatly from simply being plant-based… this lifestyle is not usually based on the welfare of animals.

Plant-based lifestyle usually pertains to a healthy lifestyle that includes being active and only eating foods that originate from plants. Even though "veganism" and "plant-based" are often interchangeable terms and most people do not know the difference. A plant-based eater is specifically concerned for their health and how they can better it.

The benefits of going plant-based range from a healthy, glowing complexion to reducing the risk of developing cancer.

According to Dr. David Katz, a practicing physician, and researcher at Yale Universities Prevention and Research Center, "A diet of minimally processed foods close to nature, predominantly plants, is decisively associated with health promotion and disease prevention." Plant-based diets are a surefire way to make sure you get all your vitamins and nutrients. If you plan your meals out properly and are willing to try the same foods in a new way, there's no reason why you should be vitamin-deficient (DISCLAIMER: This is not including chronic health problem where you have difficulties absorbing certain vitamins)

When you try to consume more wholesome foods like fruits, vegetables, whole grains, other complex carbohydrates, beans, legumes, nuts, seeds, and lots of water, you are allowing yourself fewer health problems. You are more likely to lose unnecessary weight, and you will have a significantly lower risk of heart disease. Eating less meat will reduce your risk of stroke, cardiovascular problems, and diabetes. Your blood pressure will be more regulated due to regular consumption of whole grains, Omega fatty acids, potassium, and less intake of sodium.

You will be able to manage your blood sugar by regularly consuming foods high in fiber. Fiber slows down the absorption of sugars in your bloodstream and keeps you full longer. Fiber-dense foods balance out your cortisol levels, which in turn will make you less stressed out. Also, when you switch to plant-based food, you will reduce your risk of developing cancer, like breast or colon. Inflammation may also subside; if you have arthritis, studies show that when you cut out dairy and meat from your diet, your arthritic symptoms can improve and reduce flare-ups. There are almost too many benefits to count, and way too many to list. The only way to see the broad spectrum of these benefits is to see for yourself.

Chapter Two:

Clinical Studies: Science-Backed Proof

A 2011 study[1,2,3] from Canada found 62.1% of Canadians to be overweight and 25.4% of the population to be obese. This study found vegans and vegetarians, regardless of gender, age, or location, to make up less than 6% of the obese/overweight population. Did you know that dietary cholesterol only comes from meat, fish, eggs, and milk? The same study found vegans to have significantly lower levels of cholesterol in their blood... which means a plant-based diet will not put you at risk to have clogged arteries or heart disease.

---

[1] Public Health Agency of Canada [website] Obesity in Canada: prevalence among adults. Ottawa, ON: Public Health Agency of Canada; 2011. Available from: **www.phac-aspc.gc.ca/hp-ps/hl-mvs/oic-oac/adult-eng.php**. Accessed 2018 May 14.
From <*https://www.ncbi.nlm.nih.gov/pmc/articles/PMC5638464/*>

[2] Statistics Canada [website] Body mass index of Canadian children and youth, 2009 to 2011. Ottawa, ON: Statistics Canada; 2013. Available from: **www.statcan.gc.ca/pub/82-625-x/2012001/article/11712-eng.htm**. Accessed 2018 May 12
From <*https://www.ncbi.nlm.nih.gov/pmc/articles/PMC5638464/*>

[3] Statistics Canada [website] Body composition of Canadian adults, 2009 to 2011. Ottawa, ON: Statistics Canada; 2013. Available from: **www.statcan.gc.ca/pub/82-625-x/2012001/article/11708-eng.htm**. Accessed 2018 May 12.
From <*https://www.ncbi.nlm.nih.gov/pmc/articles/PMC5638464/*>

Type 2 diabetes and cancer are both prevalent diseases of people who regularly consume animal products.

In 2015, the World Health Organization (W. H. O.) found evidence[4] linking red and processed meat consumption to colorectal cancer. This study has also found overwhelming evidence to classify processed meats such as sausages, bacon, ham, beef jerky, corned beef, smoked, fermented, and cured meats, as a group 1 carcinogen. The Academy of Nutrition and Dietetics stated that a vegan diet (when properly planned) could provide the prevention and treatment of many diseases and ailments-- it can be perfect for any person in any stage of life, including pregnancy, infancy, and athletic.

Aside from how animal products affect our health, maintenance of livestock has quite a negative impact on the Earth as well. The consumption of animal products uses an astonishing and disturbing amount of earthly resources. 60 Billion animals, per annum, are used

---

[4] World Health Organization [website] Carcinogenicity of consumption of red processed meat Lancet. Oncol. 2015 Dec; 16(16):1599-600.

to feed the human population. Livestock production is responsible for 18 % of the greenhouse gas emissions. That is more than all the vehicles on earth emit into the ozone layer. To produce a kilogram (2.2 pounds) of beef, it requires seventy times the amount of land required to produce the same amount of weight in vegetables. The amount of all irrigation water[5], the amount that is used to produce livestock is calculated to increase from 15% to 50% by 2025.

Another study[6] on people with rheumatoid arthritis, published in the journal of the American Dietetic Association in 2010, stated that when you switch to a plant-based diet, you will reduce your joint inflammation. There were significant improvements in joint tenderness, duration of stiffness in the morning, and better grip strength. Vitamins B-12 and D, Calcium, and Essential Fatty-Acids are essential for bone health. Fatty Acids are commonly found in olive and canola oils, chia, flax, and hemp seeds.

---

[5] A global assessment of the water footprint of farm animal products. 2012;15(3): 401-15. Epub 2012 Jan 24.

[6] A study done on vegan and vegetarian diets about joint health, *Journal of the American Dietetic Association, 2010.*

From < https://www.arthritis.org/living-with-arthritis/arthritis-diet/anti-inflammatory/vegan-and-vegetarian-diets.php>

A study[7] from Massachusetts General Hospital associates high consumption levels of animal protein in the human diet with higher mortality rates. The longest study of the effects of different sources of proteins, like processed and even unprocessed red meats versus plant-based, found trends in plant-based proteins and lower risk of mortality. There is a suggestion to replace some proteins with carbohydrates—which produces some health benefits, like weight management, reduced blood pressure, and other cardiovascular issues. This study stated that consuming more plant-sourced protein will help you have healthier well-being.

Apparently, going plant-based will save trillions of dollars, millions of lives, and very possibly the Earth. A study[8] done at Oxford University compared three scenarios pertaining to veganism:

---

[7] Edward Giovannucci et al. **Association of Animal and Plant Protein Intake With All-Cause and Cause-Specific Mortality.** *JAMA Internal Medicine*, 2016 DOI: 10.1001/jamainternmed.2016.4182

[8] **Analysis and valuation of the health and climate change cobenefits of dietary change**

Marco Springmann, H. Charles J. Godfray, Mike Rayner, and Peter Scarborough

PNAS April 12, 2016. 113 (15) 4146-4151; published ahead of print March 21, 2016.

https://doi.org/10.1073/pnas.1523119113

Researchers compared the effects of veganism and global mortality rates, greenhouse gas emissions, and health from an economic standpoint. A world-wide adoption of a plant-based diet predicted to prevent 8.1 million deaths per annum and reduce deaths from all causes by 10% by 2050. Adopting a plant-based diet will reduce food-related greenhouse gases by 70% by 2050.

Also, going plant-based is projected to save $1067 billion USD a year in costs related to health care. Going plant-based could literally save the world. This study is basically saying that the consumption of animal products causes an obscene amount of health problems.

Chapter Three:

Basic Four-Week Meal Plan

(also, an explanation of some vital vitamins)

(The following meal plan is not designed for weight loss or to build muscle. It is not a low-fat meal plan although you may take out or add any of the ingredients as you see fit. This is not a low-carb meal plan, you can always add more produce. Also, this is not a super-high protein plan meant for pregnant women or athletes. If you are either of these, I suggest adding more protein.)

Breakfast is absolutely the most important meal of the day. You fast for about eight hours while you sleep and when you wake up your blood sugar will be low. Even though you may not be hungry, it is important to get a little something in your stomach for fuel for your body. Your first meal should consist of protein-dense, high-fiber ingredients. These two will help keep you full and energized for the day ahead. Eating five or six small meals throughout the day will give you the boosts you need to not crash hallway through your workload. Drinking lots of water is equally important. Sometimes dehydration will mask itself as hunger.

There are a few nutrients and vitamins that will most likely come up in conversation a lot as a plant-based eater; These include vitamin D, Iron, Protein, and B12.

Vitamin D: Required to be able to absorb calcium properly. Ultimately, the best way to get Vitamin D into your system is through sunlight. Every living thing needs sunlight since it is vital for life to exist. It only takes about five to thirty minutes of sunlight twice a week for us to be able to get all the Vitamin D we need. Many plant-based milks and cereals are fortified with vitamin D. Mushrooms are naturally loaded with vitamin D. The best way to get vitamin D is by going outside and soaking up some sun. A plus side to this is the sun keeps depression at bay.

B-12: When it comes to a plant-based diet, B-12 is hard to come by in food…naturally. It is in soil, and I also produced by the bacteria in your gut, so unless you do not want to wash your produce, the best way to get your B-12 is probably through a daily supplement. Since the oral bioavailability is relatively low, try to find one with a relatively high level of a daily value percentage.

Five sources of B12 include:
1. Most plant-based milks are fortified with B12
2. The same goes for most cereals
3. Plant-based butter spreads
4. Nutritional yeast
5. Nori (seaweed)

<u>**Protein**</u>: The recommended amount of protein for the average woman is approximately 52 grams per day and for the average man, 63 grams per day. There is protein in almost everything a plant-based eater regularly consumes. Despite the controversy, protein is one of the most easily obtainable of the nutrients. Vegetables, fruits, beans, whole grains, legumes, nuts, and seeds sometimes have just some, and others have quite a bit of protein. The typical American diet has almost too much protein. Unless you are pregnant or athletic, you

really do not need as much protein as you would think. Diets high in protein tend to increase chances of osteoporosis and kidney disease.

The top 12 food that contains the highest levels of protein are:
1. Black Beans
2. Tofu
3. Nuts
4. Tempeh
5. Chickpeas
6. Broccoli
7. Quinoa
8. Lentils
9. Potatoes
10. Mushrooms
11. Plant-based milk
12. Plant-based yogurt

<u>Iron:</u> Even though iron is the most common nutrient to be deficient in human. When you are a plant-eater, getting plenty of iron into your system is easier than you would imagine. If you pair it with some form of vitamin C, you will not have any problems with anemia; Vitamin C helps your body absorb iron.

Here are the top ten sources of iron:
1. Tomato Paste
2. White Beans
3. Cooked Soybeans
4. Lentils
5. Dried Apricots

6. Spirulina
7. Spinach
8. Quinoa
9. Blackstrap Molasses
10. Prune Juice

Here is a basic Four-Week Meal Plan with recipes from all different sources. If you are not sure of how to make the recipe, there are many different variations from Minimalist Baker, Forks Over Knives, YouTube, or Eat This Much online. It is relatively simple to follow, and there is no right way to go about this plan.

WEEK 1	Breakfast	Snack	Lunch	Snack	Dinner
Monday	Oatmeal with raspberries blueberries chia seeds cinnamon almonds	Blue-Corn Chips, Black Bean Hummus	Jambalaya with Bell Peppers, Chickpeas	Fresh Fruit	Soup: Potatoes, onions, carrots, veggie broth, bay leaf, olive oil, salt, and pepper
Tuesday	Bananas with plant milk and cinnamon	Fruit, Mixed Nuts	Peanut Butter, Banana and Chia seed sandwich	Apple and Broccoli salad with Olive oil, Lemon juice, Salt, and peppercorn dressing	Rice and Black Bean burrito. Add tomatoes, spinach, salsa, avocado.
Wednesday	Oatmeal	Pretzels, carrots, celery, and peanut butter	Spaghetti with Pasta Sauce of your choice	Pretzels and Orange Juice	Quinoa Stuffed Bell Peppers
Thursday	Coconut yogurt with granola	Chips with Hummus	Whole Wheat bagel with almond butter	Apple and Broccoli Salad	Black Bean Burgers

			and Banana		
Friday	Smoothie: Banana, Spinach, blueberries, Hemp Seeds	Pretzels and Orange	Whole wheat toast with cacao and almond butter spread with Berries	Mixed nuts and fruit	Rice and Veggie soup
Saturday	Oatmeal	Chia, Banana, Almond Butter Wrap	Jambalaya with chickpeas and steamed veggies	Pretzels and Orange	Spaghetti
Sunday	Yogurt and granola	Hummus and chips	Peanut Butter and Jelly Sandwich with fruit	Fresh fruit and steamed veggies	Burritos with Walnut Meat

WEEK 2	Breakfast	Snack	Lunch	Snack	Dinner
Monday	Oatmeal	Apples and peanut butter	Pad Thai	Fresh fruit	Mixed Veggies with Brown Rice and Soy Sauce
Tuesday	Cinnamon Apple Toast	Strawberries and Chocolate Almond Milk	Tomato Soup with whole wheat garlic toast	Fresh fruit and veggies	Steamed Veggies with brown rice and sweet potato fries
Wednesday	Banana Oatmeal Smoothie	Peanut Butter and Celery	Fully Loaded Salad with Balsamic Dressing	Peanut Butter and carrots	Garlic, White wine pasta with Brussel sprouts
Thursday	Granola and coconut yogurt	Fruit and Mixed nuts	Fully loaded burrito	Chocolate Banana Smoothie	Pad Thai
Friday	Overnight Oats	Strawberries and chocolate almond milk	Couscous with pine nuts and bell peppers	Tomato and hummus on rye bread	Mixed veggies with brown rice and soy sauce

Saturday	Banana Almond Butter Toast	Pretzels and Orange	Pad Thai	Mixed Nuts	Spaghetti with Spiralized Zucchini
Sunday	Overnight Oats	Yogurt and Granola	Peanut Butter and Jelly sandwich	Pretzels and Orange	Burritos

WEEK 3	Breakfast	Snack	Lunch	Snack	Dinner
Monday	Banana Oatmeal Smoothie	Spinach Salad with Carrots	Kale and Avocado Salad	Cantaloupe with granola	White Spaghetti
Tuesday	High Protein Smoothie with Granola	Peanut Butter and Celery	Avocado Pasta Sauce	Spinach and Tomato Salad	Zucchini Peanut Noodles
Wednesday	Overnight Oatmeal	Spinach and Tomato Salad	Apricot Jam and Almond Butter Sandwich	Cabbage and Carrot Juice with Granola	Sea Salt Edamame and Lemon Cous-Cous salad
Thursday	Raspberry Chia Seed Pudding and Oranges	Basic Green smoothie with Red Bell Peppers	Banana, Peanut Butter, and Raisins with Peanut Butter and Celery	Mixed Nuts	White Spaghetti
Friday	Oatmeal and Apples with Granola	Celery and Hummus	Hummus Pocket Sandwich	Sliced Cucumber and Avocado	Fresh Tomato Pasta, Green beans with olive oil
Saturday	Chocolate milk with oatmeal,	Cantaloupe and Red Pepper	Carrot, Hummus, and avocado	Peanut Butter and Celery	Burritos

	raisins, and dates	and Hummus			
Sunday	Blueberry, Almond Butter protein smoothie	Peanut Butter and Celery	Avocado Pasta Sauce	Cucumber and Tomato toss with Granola	Sweet Potato noodles, Cashew Sauce and Brussel Sprouts

WEEK 4	Breakfast	Snack	Lunch	Snack	Dinner
Monday	Oatmeal with raspberries blueberries chia seeds cinnamon almonds	Blue-Corn Chips, Black Bean Hummus	Jambalaya with Bell Peppers, Chickpeas	Fresh Fruit	Soup: Potatoes, onions, carrots, veggie broth, bay leaf, olive oil, salt, and pepper
Tuesday	Bananas with plant milk and cinnamon	Fruit, Mixed Nuts	Peanut Butter, Banana and Chia seed sandwich	Apple and Broccoli salad with Olive oil, Lemon juice, Salt, and peppercorn dressing	Rice and Black Bean burrito. Add tomatoes, spinach, salsa, avocado.
Wednesday	Oatmeal	Pretzels, carrots, celery, and peanut butter	Spaghetti with Pasta Sauce of your choice	Pretzels and Orange Juice	Quinoa Stuffed Bell Peppers
Thursday	Coconut yogurt with granola	Chips with Hummus	Whole Wheat bagel with almond butter and Banana	Apple and Broccoli Salad	Black Bean Burgers

Day	Breakfast	Snack	Lunch	Snack	Dinner
Friday	Smoothie: Banana, Spinach, blueberries, Hemp Seeds	Pretzels and Orange	Whole wheat toast with cacao and almond butter spread with Berries	Mixed nuts and fruit	Rice and Veggie soup
Saturday	Oatmeal	Chia, Banana, Almond Butter Wrap	Jambalaya, chickpeas, steamed veggies	Pretzels and Orange	Spaghetti
Sunday	Yogurt and granola	Hummus and chips	Peanut Butter and Jelly Sandwich with fruit	Fresh fruit and steamed veggies	Burritos with Walnut Meat

PART 2

Chapter 1:

Obesity and the Standard American Diet

The Obesity Epidemic

There is no question that America is facing an obesity epidemic. An epidemic is a medical crisis that affects large parts of a population. With approximately eighty million adults and fifteen million children dealing with obesity, it has become one of the biggest health concerns today.

There is much more to obesity than being fat because obesity leads to many health problems. It is often correlated with high levels of blood sugar and insulin resistance, which, left unchecked, lead to type 2 diabetes. Excess fat in the abdominal area puts extra strain on the lumbar spine; in fact, just ten extra pounds of abdominal fat creates the equivalent of a hundred pounds of pressure on the spine. For this reason, obese people tend to suffer from back pain, sometimes to the extent that their daily routines and quality of life are affected. Extra fat places strain on the skeleton, leading many obese people to suffer from joint problems, particularly in the ankles, which bear most of the body's weight. The excess fat can build up in the blood vessels and visceral organs, leading to problems such as cardiovascular disease (including high blood pressure, heart attack, stroke, coronary artery disease, and congestive heart failure), respiratory difficulty, and fatty liver disease (which can mimic the effects of long-term alcohol abuse). Obesity can lead to hormonal disruptions, which can cause problems such as acne, polycystic ovary syndrome (PCOS) in women, and metabolic syndrome (a condition in which the body's ability to carry out its basic functions is compromised). Obese people are also more prone to sleep problems, such as sleep apnea, which occurs when the airway becomes partially blocked, causing the person to consistently wake up throughout the night. In addition to the physical problems, people who are obese also tend to struggle with emotional issues. These include challenges with self-esteem, body image, and social anxiety. Clearly, obesity is a problem that needs to be addressed and taken seriously.

While other components, such as genetics or metabolic disorders, may play a role in obesity, the main culprit leading to obesity is lifestyle choices, chiefly diet and exercise. In the nineteenth and early twentieth centuries, Americans were much more active because their lifestyles required it. People who worked on farms would be up milking cows, plowing fields, baling hay, planting crops, and harvesting from sunup to sundown. Think for a minute about how much physical energy farm work consumes! In the cities, most people did not have access to automated transportation, such as cars. Therefore, they mostly walked to their destinations, including work, school, and the grocery store. Furthermore, they did not have processed foods but only fruits, vegetables, grains, dairy, nuts, and meat that came from farms.

Today, many Americans have largely sedentary lifestyles. They drive to work, take the elevator instead of walking up the stairs, sit in chairs at their desks all day, drive home, and then watch television. Instead of bringing a healthy meal from home, many go out to eat for lunch, filling their diets with processed food and lots of sugar and little fiber (even if the food is labeled as healthy). With people getting little to no fiber, the sugar gets into the bloodstream, causing a sharp rise in insulin. High levels of insulin are linked to metabolic syndrome, weight gain, hormonal imbalances (insulin itself is a hormone), and diabetes. Instead of getting burned off through exercise, the sugar goes into the body's cells — usually much, much more than the cells require — and becomes converted into fat. Years of abusing the body through poor diet choices and lack of exercise lead to disease and a marked decrease in quality of life for individuals. As a society, it leads to a crippling burden on the medical system, causing resources (personnel, research dollars, lab equipment, etc.) that could be used to research and treat other conditions (such as pediatric cancer or spinal cord injuries) to be disproportionately allocated to treat the diseases associated with obesity.

Note that the text said "the diseases associated with obesity." The modern medical system is not as interested in treating obesity, the underlying cause of many of the diseases. The fact is that you cannot medicate yourself into health. A doctor cannot prescribe a pill that will make a patient healthy. The battle against obesity begins not in the doctor's office but in the kitchen, with the foods that people eat.

Why Are We so Fat?

The number one culprit behind the unprecedented weight gain of Americans is sugar. So many of the foods that we eat contain large amounts of added sugar; this is not only referring to sweets. Things as seemingly innocent as tomato soup and salad dressing are loaded with extra sugar. Americans consume far, far too much sugar.

The Problem with Calories

The problem with calories is essentially twofold. The first problem is that many people are not able to properly use the calories that they consume. Calories are necessary for the body to be able to function optimally. Calories are units of energy, so ideally, the number of calories that you consume will determine how much energy you have. However, the situation for many people is different, as their bodies lack the necessary vitamins and minerals needed to process that energy. That is why you may feel sluggish and tired after eating a large slice of cake (following the sugar rush, of course), which is high in calories but virtually devoid of nutrients.

The second problem with calories is that most Americans consume far, far too many of them. Not only are they not only able to properly use their calories, but the excessive number indirectly leads to weight gain. Notice that this said "indirectly" leads to weight gain, as calories themselves are not the culprit. Rather, the foods that contain the inordinate number of calories are to blame. Foods that are high in calories tend to be heavily processed and devoid of nutrients and come in supersized portions. For example, a hamburger found in a kid's happy meal is actually closer to how much an adult should consume; meanwhile, the kids eat the adult-sized hamburger while the adults eat the massive Big Mac and wash it down with a milkshake. Even processed foods that are low-calorie are deceptive, as they are also devoid of nutrients, largely unsatisfying (causing many people to consume far more than one serving), and can lead to weight gain. Nutritious foods, such as fresh fruits and vegetables, grass-fed beef, and free-range poultry are not only lower in calories than processed food but also much higher in nutrients, causing you to eat less. People who eat these foods feel full sooner, are more satisfied, and are all-around healthier.

The fact is that not all calories are created equal. One gram of sugar has four calories, while one gram of fat has nine calories. Simple arithmetic says to eat foods high in sugar rather than foods high in fat. However, this overly simplistic solution overlooks how our bodies actually use calories. Processed sugar is not necessary for the body to properly function; rather, it is hugely detrimental. In addition, if sugar is not immediately burned off, it quickly turns into fat. Furthermore, sugar has consistently been proven to actually increase someone's appetite, causing the person to consume far more than he or she normally would. While fat has more calories than sugar, there are some good types of fat that your body needs to be able to function properly. These include some saturated fats (found in free-range, grass-fed, organic animal products such as milk, beef, and eggs), omega-3 fatty acids (found in eggs and nuts), and monounsaturated fat (found in nuts and avocados). The body responds to these fats in vastly different ways than it responds to the lab-created fats — such as hydrogenated oils — found in processed foods. Eating good fats causes you to feel full, leading you to actually consume fewer calories while giving your body what it needs.

All of this is to say that instead of counting calories, what you really should be doing is paying more attention to the foods that contain those calories.

The American Diet

The typical American diet relies too much on convenience, so much so that people are willing to compromise their own physical health rather than be bothered with worrying about what they are eating. Breakfast food options in many supermarkets are centered on convenience rather than nutrition: sugary cereals, Pop-tarts, frozen breakfast sandwiches, and instant oatmeal. Most of these processed options have had most of their nutritional contents removed (instant oatmeal has far less fiber and other nutrients than steel-cut oats) and lots of sugar added. They are also devoid of fresh fruit (despite many of the claims on packages). Sadly, many people consume these products rather than making a nutritious breakfast that includes fresh fruit and protein. When office workers go out to lunch every day rather than bringing a healthy, pre-packed lunch from home, the reason is usually because going to a restaurant is more convenient than waking up fifteen minutes earlier. Going to a drive-through after a long day of work is so much more convenient than preparing a nutritious meal from scratch.

The result of all this convenience is way, way too many carbs, too much sodium, and too much unhealthy fat, such as hydrogenated oils, and far too few nutrients, such as vitamins, minerals, and fiber. Some people think that they can correct this imbalance by taking a multivitamin and fiber supplement every morning. However, the quality of the vitamins and minerals in supplements is of lower quality than of those found in fresh food, and they don't exist in the natural combination that our bodies require for optimal processing. In fact, the body only absorbs about ten to twenty percent of the nutrients found in a multivitamin. Fiber supplements can be of assistance, especially to people who are elderly but cannot produce all the benefits of including fiber in the diet throughout the day. Those benefits include lower levels of blood sugar and insulin and feeling full for longer.

What may be shocking to many people is that a lot of Americans are malnourished! This type of malnourishment is not the result of an inadequate amount of food but by poor food choices. Furthermore, excessive sugar actually reduces the body's ability to absorb the nutrients that it does receive. Many Americans have critically low levels of crucial vitamins such as D, K, and the B complex, which prohibit their bodies from being able to function optimally. This is yet another reason why so many people are sick.

Abdominal Fat Problem: Fastest Place to Lose Weight

One of the most dangerous places for the body to store fat is in the abdominal area; excess abdominal fat is so dangerous that it is actually a predictor of conditions such as heart disease and type 2 diabetes. The good news is that abdominal fat is the easiest type to lose. You don't have to do crunches or sit-ups to lose it; rather, you simply need to change your diet.

Abdominal fat is created by poor diet choices, such as excessive sugar, alcohol, and processed foods that contain unhealthy fats. In order to start losing it, eat foods that are low in sugar and other refined carbs, high in fiber, and high in protein. Examples include fresh fruits and vegetables, homemade soups and stews, and nuts and seeds. To further fight the belly bulge, rather than doing abdominal exercises, the best exercise to do is cardio, such as brisk walking and swimming.

Problems and Trappings of a High-Carb Diet

Americans consume far, far too much sugar and other refined carbs. Even though carbs are lower in calories than fats, they lead to weight gain. Refined carbs actually "flip a switch" inside the brain that signals that you need to keep eating more carbs. Furthermore, a few hours afterward, you may have a craving to eat more carbs. As a result, you end up consuming an excessive amount of empty calories instead of giving your body the nutrition that it needs.

In summary, Americans are facing an unprecedented health crisis brought on not by lack of food, but by an overabundance of food. Americans are consuming far too many calories, but are actually malnourished because the calories that they consume are not filled with the nutrients that they need for their bodies to function properly. Furthermore, too many Americans lack an understanding of what calories really are and what our bodies need in order to use them as energy. As a result, much of the population is fat and sick.

Chapter 2:

Knowledge About Proper Nutrition

What Causes High Blood Sugar and High Blood Pressure?

High blood sugar exists when the bloodstream is filled with more sugar than it can process. When sugar enters the bloodstream, insulin is secreted by the pancreas to enable the body's cells to absorb the sugar and use it for energy. However, if there is more sugar in the bloodstream than the cells need, it builds up and insulin levels remain high. Over time, high insulin levels cause the cells to stop responding to it as efficiently, so more is required for them to absorb the sugar from the blood. If this is not corrected, the result can be insulin resistance. Insulin resistance will cause blood sugar levels to remain high, no matter how much insulin is secreted. If left untreated, diabetes can ensue.

The cause of high blood sugar is simple: too much sugar and not enough fiber in the diet. When sugar is consumed with fiber — for example, in fresh fruit, which contains sugar but also contains fiber — it released into the bloodstream more slowly, giving the body time to allow the cells to absorb it. However, when sugar is consumed without any fiber — for example, in a soda or piece of cake — it jets into the bloodstream, causing blood sugar levels to rise.

Blood pressure refers to the force of blood pressing against the walls of blood vessels; high blood pressure means that the blood is pressing too hard, which, over time, can cause damage to the cardiovascular system. The blood vessels can become stiff and hard, a sometimes fatal condition referred to as atherosclerosis. Poor diet choices are also behind many cases of high blood pressure. While there is a genetic component for *some* cases of high blood pressure, it is more often than not linked to the typical American diet. Rather than being linked to excessive sugar intake, high blood pressure seems to be more associated with excessive salt (most processed foods have very high levels of sodium) and bad fats, such as hydrogenated oils.

Lectins and Why They Are Bad

Lectins are proteins that bind to both cell membranes and sugar. They are found in nearly all plants and animals because they help cells communicate with each other. However, they can be very dangerous. One reason why is that some lectins are extremely toxic. For example, ricin, a toxin that is fatal in extremely small amounts, is derived from the lectins found in the castor bean.

Another reason why lectins are so dangerous is that they cause inflammation. Inflammation is one of the body's natural defenses against infection and other foreign invaders. However, over time, inflammation can lead to heart disease, hormonal disruptions, aches and pains, and a host of other problems. In addition, lectins can contribute to leaky gut syndrome, something that will be explained in detail in Chapter 7.

Lectins are found in nearly all of the foods that we consume. However, the biggest culprits include white potatoes, eggplant, beans, and dairy. Dairy poses a double danger because it is actually designed to penetrate the lining of the intestine, the cause of the leaky gut syndrome. These seemingly healthy foods should be avoided at all costs.

In summary, many Americans struggle with high blood sugar and high blood pressure. However, they do not understand how their poor diets and lifestyle choices are actually creating these problems. High blood sugar and high blood pressure are caused by consuming sugary processed food; high blood pressure is also the result of eating too much meat. These conditions can actually be reversed by changing eating patterns. In addition, lectins are proteins found in nearly all foods but are toxic, especially when consumed in large amounts. While plant-based foods should be consumed in favor of processed foods and meat, special care should be taken to avoid lectins.

CHAPTER 3: LACK OF EXERCISE

Have you ever bought a gym membership at the beginning of the year? Gyms tend to heavily discount their memberships to entice the hordes of people making New Year's resolutions about getting fit and losing weight. They aren't taking a risk by offering their product/service at a rate that is too low because they know that within a month, most of the people who bought a membership will forget that they even have it. Most of those gym memberships will be used for a few weeks before being forgotten for the rest of the year.

This highlights the fact that Americans get far too little exercise. Our lifestyles have become quite sedentary, exemplified by the long hours that we sit at desks using computers (both at work and at home) and how much time we spend watching television. While for our ancestors' exercise was built into their daily routines, through activities such as hunting, farming, and walking long distances, we don't really need to exercise to get through the day. There are exceptions, such as occupations that require people to be on their feet constantly or those that involve heavy labor. However, for the most part, we are able to get through our lives just fine without any exercise. This lack of exercise is taking a huge toll on the nation's health. Not only are we consuming far too much sugar and processed foods, but we are not burning off any of those excessive calories.

The benefits of exercise beyond burning calories are tremendous. Exercise releases endorphins, which boost the mood; therefore, exercise is nature's own antidepressant. Chronic stress, something that many Americans struggle with (some without even realizing it, because stress has become such a normal part of life), causes hormones such as cortisol and adrenaline to be released into the bloodstream. High levels of cortisol are known to lead to weight gain, especially in the abdominal area. Exercise, however, burns off cortisol and other hormones that, over time, can cause damage. Exercise helps people sleep better at night, improves heart health, regulates and even decreases appetite, produces more mental clarity, lowers blood pressure, and burns off excessive blood sugar. With all of these benefits, in addition to burning calories, it is a wonder that exercise is not prescribed more than medication!

In summary, the benefits of exercise cannot be overstated. It increases bone and muscle strength, strengthens the heart, improves blood flow, and boosts mood. However, too many Americans lead largely sedentary lives that are practically devoid of exercise. As a result, their bodies are not able to function properly and they are chronically lethargic and fatigued. Instead of dealing with the root of the problem — lack of exercise — many opt for expensive and dangerous medications.

Chapter 4:

Downfall of Medication

When is the last time you saw a commercial or online advertisement about lawsuits for people who took a certain medication and experienced dangerous side effects? When is the last time you saw a commercial or online advertisement for a particular medication, and in the fine print was a list of dozens of harmful side effects, some of which could be life-threatening? Up until 1985, advertising prescription medications directly to consumers rather than to doctors was illegal. However, nowadays our media is inundated with ads for prescription medications, and as a society, we have become fixated on the idea that a pill can cure most, if not all, of our ailments.

What Medication Does to Your Body

The reality is that while medication can alleviate some symptoms and be very beneficial in critical cases, it can also be very damaging to the body. This section will look at different types of medication and the harm that they can cause.

Antidepressants. Approximately 10% of the US population is on antidepressants, and they are the third most prescribed category of medication. Most antidepressants work by preventing neurons from reabsorbing the hormone serotonin, the "feel-good" hormone. This raises overall serotonin levels, but over time, causes an imbalance of serotonin inside and outside of neurons. Because serotonin does more than elevating mood (it also aids in the growth and death of neurons, digestion, reproduction, and blood clotting), imbalanced levels can lead to problems such as digestive problems (including abdominal bleeding), sexual dysfunction, and sleep disturbances. Furthermore, after prolonged use (even just a few months), the brain begins to push back after the effects of the drug in order to restore the proper balance of serotonin. This can lead to a full-blown relapse of depression, even while people are still taking the medication. Commonly, doctors will either increase the dose or switch patients to a stronger antidepressant without appreciating that the brain itself is working against the drug.

Painkillers. Painkillers are usually taken in the form of over-the-counter medication to alleviate discomfort associated with aches and pains, including menstrual cramps and arthritis. While many people are aware of the dangers of narcotic painkillers, even OTC ones are harmful. They work by preventing nerves from being able to carry out their functions, namely, to transmit messages from different parts of the body to the brain. Long-term use can actually lead to nerve damage. In addition, they are harmful to the liver and can cause stomach bleeding, which can be fatal.

Antibiotics. Antibiotics are commonly prescribed to treat bacterial infections, such as respiratory infections. They work by killing off the bacteria inside the body. However, the body naturally contains good bacteria, including approximately five pounds of it in the gut alone! This gut bacteria are known as the microbiome and are essential to carrying out many vital functions, including absorption of nutrients and regulation of hormones. Because antibiotics are indiscriminate in the bacteria that they kill, they devastate the microbiome and therefore disrupt many of the body's natural processes.

In addition, strains of bacteria are becoming resistant to antibiotics. This is because as a nation, we have become so dependent on medications, believing that a pill can fix all of our health problems, that we have overused antibiotics. Some patients are so insistent on getting medicated for whatever ailments they have that they are prescribed antibiotics for viruses, such as colds, something that antibiotics are powerless against. In response, the bacteria develop defenses to protect them from the antibiotics. The result is that new and difficult-to-treat diseases, such as MRSA, are becoming increasingly common.

Ultimately, medication is able to alleviate the symptoms of the disease, but it is not able to cure the overall dysfunction that led to the problem. Statins can lower cholesterol, but they cannot fix the cause of high cholesterol: poor diet and lack of exercise. Antibiotics can fight off foreign invaders that lead to infection, but they cannot heal the body so that it is able to defend itself through its natural mechanisms without antibiotics. If you want to actually address the cause of your symptoms rather than become a revolving-door patient, you need to fix and change your diet.

In summary, there is no benefit that medication can provide that adequate nutrition and exercise cannot provide, but without the damaging side effects. Exercise is more effective at treating depression and anxiety than antidepressants and other mood-enhancing medications. Having an optimized microbiome in the gut, fed with plenty of high-fiber fruits, vegetables, and probiotics, cannot only treat infections better than antibiotics but can eliminate the pathogens before they even take hold. Our lifestyles are what have made us sick, and medication cannot fix a lifestyle problem. Medications are dangerous and produce side effects that can pose long-term health risks. A healthy plant-based diet, however, can replace the need for medication.

CHAPTER 5:

CASE STUDIES OF PLACES WITH THE HIGHEST LONGEVITY

Despite its reputation for being wealthy and prosperous, the United States actually ranks number 50 in the world in terms of life expectancy, with Americans living an average of just over 78 years. Countries that fare better have several things in common, including social factors that cause people to lead healthier lifestyles. The world's highest life expectancy — nearly 90 years — is found in Monaco, which also has the world's highest population of millionaires and billionaires. Since most of the rest of us can't afford the kind of lifestyle that may contribute to the high longevity of residents of Monaco, that and other small, wealthy states will be disregarded.

Okinawa, Japan. The Japanese inhabitants of the island of Okinawa eat a low-fat diet that largely consists of fish, tofu, seaweed, and vegetables. Many of them actually only consume 1200 calories a day; however, their life expectancy is approximately 87 years, three years longer than their other Japanese compatriots. In fact, Okinawa has five times as many centenarians as the rest of Japan! Many Okinawans remain healthy until the end of their lives, and those who are 80 years old may have bodies that more closely resemble that of someone in his or her forties or fifties.

Loma Linda, California. Loma Linda is a small town of about 25,000 people, about sixty miles from Los Angeles. It is the center of the Seventh-Day Adventist Church, which advocates a plant-based diet and strongly discourages smoking. The different lifestyle habits of the church's members may be what contributes to the fact that its residents enjoy a life expectancy of about 85 years, as compared to the rest of the United States, which is only about 78 years.

Iceland. The small Nordic country of Iceland has an average life expectancy of just under 83 years, the highest in Europe. It also has exceptionally low infant mortality. These results can be at least partially attributed to the clean energy used to provide for the nation's power needs. However, they can also be attributed to the traditional diet of Iceland, which is high in fish, and a culture that promotes being physically active, especially outdoors.

In summary, cultures that promote the highest rates of longevity have several things in common. The people tend to be more active than in other parts of the world, thereby reaping the myriad benefits of exercise. Their diets are low in meat and other animal products and high in fruits and vegetables.

Chapter 6:

Who This Book Is For

If you are struggling with any health problems, even those that may be genetic, then this book is for you. This chapter will look at what the plant-based diet can do for many common health problems.

Autoimmune disease. An autoimmune disease results when the body's immune system believes that healthy cells are foreign invaders and attacks them as such. Examples of autoimmune diseases include Crohn's, rheumatoid arthritis, and multiple sclerosis. Chronic inflammation is believed to be one of the causes; in fact, it is the culprit behind many chronic diseases. Inflammation is triggered by foods high in sugar and excessive consumption of meat, especially processed meat. Eating a diet mostly from plants results not only in less inflammation but a reversal of the damage caused by long-term inflammation! Many people with autoimmune diseases who have switched to a plant-based diet have noticed not only that their symptoms are largely alleviated but also that the disease itself becomes reversed.

Irritable bowel syndrome (IBS). IBS is a condition that affects as much as 15% of the American population; it results in intestinal dysfunction, including cramping, bloating, diarrhea, abdominal pain, gas, and constipation. Eating a plant-based diet has proven to considerably help people with IBS. Fresh fruits and vegetables are high in prebiotics, which promote a healthy environment for the good bacteria that make up the colon's microbiome. Proper functioning of the microbiome is essential to bowel health, as well as the health of the rest of the body.

Brain fog. Brain fog, or a generalized lack of clarity, can be substantially helped by eating a plant-based diet. When your body is out of whack, usually caused by poor diet choices and lack of exercise, your mood and thinking can be dramatically affected. Giving your body the nutrition that it needs will ameliorate most, if not all of the problems that are contributing to fuzzy and clouded thinking as well as a depressed mood.

Arthritis. Arthritis, a painful joint condition, is caused largely by chronic inflammation in the joints. As previously stated, inflammation is caused by eating a diet high in refined carbs, especially sugars, and meat, especially processed meat. However, a plant-based diet will not only bring down inflammation but can actually reduce the damage caused by long-term chronic inflammation.

High blood pressure. Eating a lot of salt, as part of a diet high in processed food and low in fruits and vegetables, is the primary contributing factor to high blood pressure. Studies have shown that reduced consumption of meat — consuming only one or two servings a week — resulted in most participants, blood pressure was reduced by about 25%. This result was achieved without a drug supplement. Going to a full vegetarian diet reduced blood pressure by up to 40%.

High cholesterol. Cholesterol is found exclusively in animal products. Plants on their own do not produce cholesterol. Our bodies naturally produce some cholesterol, which is generally considered to be of the beneficial type. However, high consumption of meat and products derived from animals, results in high levels of bad cholesterol, which can lead to heart disease and other problems. Switching to a plant-based diet will naturally lower your cholesterol levels simply because you won't be consuming nearly as much.

Heart disease. The reason that heart disease is the primary cause of death in America is because of poor diets and lack of exercise. Americans fill their days with sedentary activities and lots of processed, sugary foods that are also high in sodium. Eating much less meat, especially red meat, eliminating sugar and processed food, and eating mostly vegetable- and fruit-based foods have been shown to dramatically lower rates of heart disease and even reverse it in people who already suffer from it.

Acid reflux. Acid reflux is a condition in which stomach acid is propelled upwards into the esophagus, causing a burning sensation. While one out of five Americans suffers from acid reflux, in rural African villages, the risk was only one in one thousand, making it virtually unheard of. Most foods in the American diet are highly acidic, thereby contributing to the symptoms. However, plant-based foods are more alkaline, or basic, and bases neutralize acids.

Overweight or obese. People who are overweight or obese and switch to a plant-based diet, rather than relying on low-calorie processed foods, lose much more weight. Feeding your body what it needs, instead of what tastes better, results in feelings of fullness, satiation, and fewer calories consumed. Further, because those calories are useful and used efficiently by the body, people have more energy and are able to exercise more.

Those who want to look healthier. When people want to brighten their complexions, look younger, and generally look healthier, they usually go to a salon for an expensive treatment or buy a skin cream. While these procedures may make people look healthier, true health comes from the inside and is reflected in the outer appearance. In other words, when people are healthy on the inside, they look healthy on the outside.

Reverse aging. Processed foods loaded with chemicals and sugar, along with large amounts of meat and dairy, cause our bodies to age faster. However, a plant-based diet can actually reverse some of the signs and symptoms of aging. While it can't reverse the aging process, it can slow it down. Telomeres are structures at the end of our cells' DNA that keep the double-helix structure from unwinding. Every time a cell divides, the telomere is weakened, leading to the effects of aging. Telomerase is an enzyme that helps rebuild telomeres, and a plant-based diet is linked with stronger telomerase activity. What this means is that a plant-based diet can help reverse some of the effects of aging and even slow the aging process.

In summary, many of the diseases that plague modern society are the direct result of poor lifestyle choices. Changing the way that we eat can reverse and even eliminate not only short-term infections and other acute diseases but also chronic diseases, as well. All of this is to say that whoever you are, whatever health problems you may be struggling with, the plant-based miracle diet is for you.

Chapter 7:

Leaky Gut Syndrome

What is Leaky Gut Syndrome?

Leaky gut syndrome, like obesity, is becoming a national epidemic due to poor foot choices by much of the American population. The leaky gut syndrome has also been called intestinal hyperpermeability. The walls of the intestine are porous so that the nutrients in food can be absorbed into the bloodstream. However, in leaky gut, they become excessively porous, to the point that larger portions of undigested food, including waste and toxins, to enter the bloodstream. In response, the body begins to attack the foreign invaders. The liver works hard to filter out all of the food macromolecules but is unable to keep up with their constant flow into the bloodstream. The immune system then kicks in and attacks the macromolecules. They are then absorbed into the body's tissues, resulting in inflammation. As you have already seen, chronic inflammation is at the root of many diseases. Instead of carrying out its normal functions, such as filtering the blood and reducing inflammation, your body will actually go to war against itself, which can result in autoimmune disease.

Fungus Theory

Candida is a fungus that can live in your intestines; one theory about the origin of leaky gut syndrome is that it is the result of an overgrowth of candida. The theory states when a candida yeast infection grows unchecked, the fungus grows "roots" into the walls of the intestines. The wall of the intestine becomes overly porous, allowing large particles of undigested food to pass into the bloodstream.

Plant Protein

Protein from some plant sources, such as soy and wheat (wheat protein is gluten), should be avoided at all costs, as they are considered to be "anti-nutrients." Celiac disease, or gluten intolerance, is related to the leaky gut syndrome in that consuming gluten can actually lead to a 70% increase in intestinal permeability. Soy protein is just as bad; not only is 90% of soy genetically modified (which leads to a host of other problems) but on a molecular level, it mimics gluten. As a result, soy protein can also dramatically increase intestinal permeability.

Intestinal Irritants

Intestinal irritants can be behind many cases of leaky gut syndrome. There is no universal list of intestinal irritants; rather, the foods that should be avoided are, to some extent, particular to the individual. However, some of the most common culprits are caffeine, wheat (specifically, the gluten found in wheat), sugar, and soy. When foods that are intestinal irritants to you enter the bowel, they can pass through the bowel membrane and into the bloodstream.

To find what foods are problematic for you, eliminate consumption of one item at a time, for two weeks, and then gradually reintroduce it back into your diet to see what effect it has. For example, eliminate all dairy products for two weeks. Keep a journal to gauge whether you feel better or worse. At the end of two weeks, gradually begin consuming dairy again. Do you feel better or worse? If you feel worse when consuming it, dairy is probably an intestinal irritant for you.

There may be other foods that are intestinal irritants for you that are not on the general list. If you are still having problems, you may need to see a specialist to determine exactly what foods should be avoided, at least until your gut heals.

Lectin Plant Proteins

Lectins are proteins found in nearly all foods; they are produced by plants and therefore consumed by animals that eat plants. Thus, they make their way into the entire food system. Consumption of lectins cannot be avoided; however, you should try to limit them as much as possible, especially if you are dealing with leaky gut syndrome.

Lectins are problematic for leaky gut syndrome because they gravitate towards areas like the lining of the gut, where they attach themselves and cause intestinal damage. Eliminating all grains and soy, which tend to be very high in lectins, will help heal your gut. Once the lining is restored, you can gradually add back in grains that have been fermented and sprouted; these grains have smaller amounts of lectins.

Whole Grains and Resistant Starches

Whole grains are usually described as healthy. However, that is only partially true, as they may be healthier than their refined (white) counterparts in areas such as glycemic index. In fact, whole grain bread is higher in lectins than white bread because the refining process significantly reduces the amount of lectins. Consider that the grains harvested to make bread and other foods are actually the seeds of plants. If all of a plant's seeds were eaten, that plant would become extinct; therefore, nature evolved a way to prevent seeds from being eaten. Seeds have a hard shell that is lined with lectins and other anti-nutrients, to keep them from being eaten. This reason is why whole grains, even more than white grains, contribute to leaky gut syndrome.

Instead of whole grains, opt for sprouted grains. Sprouted grains have been allowed to germinate before being milled into flour, thereby eliminating the toxins contained in the shell of the seed. Sprouted grains have significantly fewer lectins but still retain the nutrient content (unlike white, refined grains). Many kinds of bread now, such as Ezekiel bread, are being made from sprouted grains.

Potatoes and beans are often heralded as "resistant starches," meaning that the starch isn't digested and the calories are not absorbed. However, potatoes, beans, and other resistant starches are high in saponin, which actually creates holes in the cells that line the intestines. Even just a small amount of the cellular damage created by saponins can prevent nutrients from being transported by the cells. Furthermore, these resistant starches contain something called protease inhibitors, which increase levels of trypsin. Trypsin is an enzyme that damages the connections between the cells that line the intestines, thereby increasing the gut's permeability.

In summary, leaky gut syndrome is one of the diseases plaguing modern society because it is caused by poor diet. It is behind many cases of inflammation, abdominal discomfort, autoimmune disease, and toxins in the blood. Leaky gut syndrome is brought on by eating foods high in lectins, including seemingly healthy whole grains and beans. It is also caused by eating genetically modified food, dairy, caffeine, and any other foods that may be particularly irritating to you as an individual.

All of this may sound like a long list of foods to be avoided. However, the plant-based miracle diet is more about increasing your palate and enjoying foods that you would never have even considered.

Chapter 8:

The Plant-Based Miracle Diet

What is the Plant-Based Miracle Diet?

Rather than being an eating plan that you stick to for a set period of time, the plant-based miracle diet is essentially a revolution of lifestyle in which permanent lifestyle changes are made. Instead of opting for eating a certain number of calories each day or getting into an exercise regimen until certain results are achieved, the plant-based miracle diet is about eliminating all processed foods eating only whole foods or those that are minimally processed.

There are three forms of the plant-based miracle diet; whichever one you decide will depend on your body type, goals, and the lifestyle changes that you are willing to make. The first form allows for some consumption of meat, as long as it is only free-range, grass-fed, and organic. Modern farming methods aim to raise animals as quickly as possible so as to create the most profit for the food company; therefore, animals raised for their meat are fed subpar food that includes unused body parts from other animals, plastic pellets, and even manure. The animals often live in unhealthy conditions, being crammed into cages that are too small and living on top of each other. They aren't able to get any exercise, and as a result of these conditions, the animals themselves are sick. To keep them from getting sick and to help them grow faster, many animals are fed a steady stream of antibiotics (most antibiotics used today are for farming). Consider that anytime you eat conventional meat, you are consuming a sick animal. That reason alone is enough to make the switch to eating only meat that is organic, grass-fed, and free range. However, the bulk of the diet consists of fruits and vegetables, and meat is eaten no more than two or three times a week.

The second form of this diet is vegetarianism, which includes the consumption of wild-caught fish (rather than farmed fish, which are subject to many of the farming methods listed above) and organic eggs from free-range chickens or other poultry. The third form of this diet is complete veganism, in which absolutely no animal products are consumed.

Choosing what works for you may be a process in which you make some lifestyle changes, such as eating more fruits and vegetables while reducing your consumption of meat until you switch to vegetarianism. You may be entirely unable or unwilling to make the switch to vegetarianism, but you make sure that all of your meat is from healthy animals rather than those raised in a factory farm. You may already be a vegetarian but want to incorporate more fruits and vegetables into your diet until you transition all the way to veganism. Whichever choice is best for you, make sure that the changes you make are ones that you can and will stick with.

In addition to a significantly reduced meat consumption, the plant-based miracle diet is, well, about eating more plant-based foods. Conventional wisdom, such as the food pyramid, says that we should aim to eat five servings of fruits and vegetables a day. This mindset sets us up for the belief that we should add fruits and vegetables into the diet that we already consume, thereby making it healthy. For example, when eating out you may decide to substitute a side salad for fries, thereby making your meal healthy. However, nothing could be further from the truth. The side salad might add one serving of vegetables to a meal loaded with hydrogenated oil, refined carbohydrates, sugar, and trans fat. It can hardly begin to offset the damaging effects of this meal.

The entire diet actually needs to be overhauled, not to make room for more fruits and vegetables, but to make plant-based foods the foundation on which the entire diet is built. Instead of ordering a side salad with a hamburger or slice of pizza, the salad should be the main dish of the meal, possibly with a small amount of meat added as a topping. Instead of eating a bowl of cereal that claims to have fruit added, the fruit should be the centerpiece of breakfast. A bowl of fruit with sprouted-grain toast and an egg would be a much healthier, plant-based option.

Because so much of the American diet is built around convenience, making the change to a plant-based diet is not just changing the foods you eat but changing your entire lifestyle. You have to change the way that you think about food. Food is not meant to be convenient or something that you eat mindlessly throughout the day. Rather, it is the source from which your body derives its health. Aristotle is credited with saying that food should be your medicine. That should be your attitude about food.

If you must have coffee in the morning, instead of stopping by Starbucks on the way to work or even filling up at the office coffee pot, make a pot of organic coffee at home (coffee has some of the highest levels of pesticides and other chemicals of any crop in the world). Instead of going out to lunch because it is easier than preparing a lunch at home, make the lifestyle changes necessary in order to either prepare your lunch the night before or wake up ten minutes earlier so that you can prepare it in the morning. Invest in a slow cooker so that healthy soups and stews can cook while you are at work, and a healthy plant-based supper will be waiting for you when you get home.

The way that you shop for groceries will have to change. If you are used to clipping coupons and buying foods that are on sale, you will have to completely change how you think about buying food. Some foods, such as conventional, factory-farm milk and wheat-based products, are subsidized by the US government to keep the prices low for consumers while still giving the farmers a profit. However, as you have seen, these foods contribute to many of the health problems that are plaguing Americans today. Instead of opting for foods that are cheap or convenient, such as microwavable frozen dinners, go first to the organic part of the produce section. By far, the bulk of what you buy should be in this section.

Other options for procuring plant-based foods include going local. Farmers markets are great places to find produce and grass-fed meat that is raised by small, local farmers. While conventional produce may be grown on the other side of the world and picked before it is ripe so that it can be shipped to the United States, the produce at a farmer's market is usually picked either that day or the day before. Because small farmers are not usually subsidized and their costs tend to be higher than those of conventional farmers, the foods found at farmer's markets can be more expensive. If you qualify for programs such as WIC, they can help offset the cost. The quality of the food and value to the local economy, rather than big agricultural corporations, make the higher cost worth it.

Besides a farmer's market, you can also see if there are any pick-your-own farms in your area. A pick-your-own farm grows the produce, but local people go in and pick it. You pay after you are finished picking; the cost is based on the weight of produce that you picked. The farmers don't weigh you before and after, so you are free to eat as much as you want while you are out picking! Going to a pick-your-own farm can be a great family outing in which children learn more about food and where it comes from while being able to procure it for themselves. It will certainly be a different type of outing than a trip to the movies or a favorite restaurant!

As you can probably see, the plant-based diet involves more than simply changing what you eat. It is changing how you think about food and, in turn, making lifestyle changes to accommodate the new mindset.

Why Should You Get on This Diet?

As previously explained, many, if not most, of the health problems facing Americans today are related directly to the foods that they eat. Refined carbohydrates, especially sugar, cause a slew of problems ranging from metabolic syndrome, weight gain, and obesity, destruction of the microbiome, to insulin resistance and diabetes. Some have been tricked into believing that they can make a healthy switch from refined carbs to whole grains, such as swapping out their white bread for whole wheat bread. However, while whole grains have a lower glycemic index than refined carbs, they are high in lectins, which can damage the wall of the intestines and lead to leaky gut syndrome. Lack of adequate vitamins and minerals due to not eating enough fruits and vegetables causes problems with immunity, blood clotting, and other disorders that are commonly associated with malnutrition.

So many of these problems can be fixed — and are getting fixed — by getting onto the plant-based diet. Eliminating all processed foods and eating only whole foods is proving across the board to have a marked effect on people's health and even curing diseases, such as diabetes and terminal cancer, that were believed to be irreversible. Furthermore, a plant-based diet leads to higher levels of energy and a better mood, leading to an overall higher quality of life.

How to Attain a Clean Diet

Most of the foods that are grown through conventional methods are "dirty." This means that not only are the methods used to grow them very destructive to the environment (large amounts of wasted water, water being contaminated by sewage, large amounts of energy needed to transport them), but they are also loaded with pesticides and other chemicals that are not safe for human consumption. Many of the pesticides that the FDA has labeled "safe" are far more dangerous to both humans and the environment than the DDT that was outlawed in 1972.

In addition to high levels of pesticides, some major biotechnical companies, such as Monsanto and Syngenta, have manufactured genetically modified seeds. GMOs are touted as having unique benefits because of the DNA that was changed, allowing them to have properties such as being resistant to drought, having higher levels of certain vitamins, or being able to withstand the stronger pesticides sprayed on them. GMOs are so ubiquitous today that unless the label on your food says that it is organic or non-GMO, you can be certain that it does contain GMOs. GMOs are very harmful to human health on two main fronts. The first is that they contain particularly high levels of the dangerous pesticide glyphosate, which is a known carcinogen. The second is that it actually changes the DNA of some human cells and the bacteria that make up the gut's microbiome. It should come as no surprise that the rise of GMOs and the rise of the leaky gut syndrome have happened simultaneously. Furthermore,

GMOs are incredibly destructive to the environment and have the potential to permanently alter the DNA of some species.

Many of these chemicals are stored in the liver, which acts as a filter. However, when the liver becomes overloaded because so many chemicals are entering our bodies, the chemicals are stored in fat cells. Because the body needs a place to store these toxins, it will refuse to get rid of excess fat cells. Losing weight can have as much to do with the chemicals in our food as with the food itself.

With this in mind, eating a plant-based diet is not enough. You need to ensure that the "healthy" whole foods that you are consuming are also clean, meaning free from these dangerous chemicals. The two ways to ensure that your food is not loaded with chemicals is to either make sure that it is labeled as GMO-free or organic or buy it locally from small farmers.

Scientific Mechanisms Behind the Plant-Based Diet

Genes are behind some of the diseases that we face. For example, some scientists have proposed that there is actually a genetic tendency for some people to gain weight easier and have a harder time losing it than other people. Some people are genetically more prone to addictive behaviors, such as smoking and overeating. Diseases such as cancer and Alzheimer's even have a genetic component! Genes are seen as an insurmountable obstacle to overcoming disease and attaining health and wellness. However, more and more studies are showing that a healthy lifestyle built around the plant-based diet can actually have more of an impact on disease, health, and well-being than genes.

In most cases, genes on their own do not cause disease (exceptions include childhood diseases such as cystic fibrosis). Rather, they predispose people to become more likely to develop a disease. For example, Mary Grace may have a gene that makes her more susceptible to developing breast cancer. All people have some number of cancerous cells in their bodies at all times, but they are usually destroyed by healthy cells that are properly functioning. Mary Grace's faulty gene may work in such a way that breast cells are more prone to turning into dangerous cancer cells, and the healthy remaining cells are less able to destroy the cancerous cells. That tendency can be either mitigated or augmented by her lifestyle. If she eats lots of damaging sugar and processed foods, her healthy cells will be even less capable of protecting her from cancerous cells. However, if she eats a diet that is based on organic, plant-based foods, she will be providing her healthy cells with the ability to fight off and destroy the cancerous cells. Furthermore, she will be giving the healthy cells the nutrients that they need to keep from mutating into cancerous cells in the first place. This example is just one way of how the plant-based miracle diet can override a person's genes and promote overall wellness.

In summary, the plant-based diet is a complete change of lifestyle, from one that is based on convenience and leads to disease, to one based on an understanding of health, well-being, and how certain foods contribute to an enhanced quality of life. It is not a list of foods that you can and can't eat, a point system, or measure of calories. You can't go to the grocery store and just buy a different brand of chips or cookies that are formulated to be compatible with this diet. Rather, you have to change how you think about food and be willing to make the necessary lifestyle changes to make whole, plant-based foods the centerpiece of your diet. These lifestyle changes include filling your shopping cart with produce rather than grains and meats, cooking meals at home (usually from scratch) instead of eating out, and eating food that is organic. The benefits produced by the plant-based diet — added years to life and life to years — make all of the effort worth it.

Chapter 9:

Benefits of the Plant-Based Miracle Diet

Stabilize Blood Sugar and Blood Pressure

High blood sugar and high blood pressure are some of the biggest health woes causing disease today. However, the plant-based miracle diet can help stabilize and even reverse the conditions.

The elimination of all processed foods means that sugar consumption is drastically reduced; most sugars come from fruits and the breakdown of sprouted grains. As natural sources of sugar, these foods also contain high levels of fiber, which slows the sugar's absorption as well as the uptake of insulin. Because less sugar is entering the bloodstream, less insulin is needed to transport it to cells for energy. Even if someone already has developed insulin resistance, meaning that increasingly high levels of insulin are required to process the sugar, consuming less sugar means that less insulin will be required. Less sugar entering the blood, coupled with that sugar being processed efficiently by insulin so that it can be used by the cells, means that excess blood sugar is completely eradicated. Over time, stabilized blood sugar can lead to insulin resistance being reversed.

Sugar is a highly addictive substance, even more addictive than some illegal drugs. For the first few weeks, you may feel the effects of sugar withdrawal, which can include headaches, lightheadedness, anxiety, depression, moodiness, and irritability. You may be tempted to say that your blood sugar is too low and you need to eat a dessert to bring it back up. However, added sugars have absolutely no health benefit. Instead, you should eat fruit (a well-made fruit salad can satisfy a sweet tooth) and sprouted grains, which will keep your blood sugar stabilized instead of causing it to spike and then plummet.

In addition to helping stabilize your blood sugar, the plant-based miracle diet can help stabilize high blood pressure. The main culprits behind high blood pressure are obesity, which causes the heart to work harder, and processed food, which contains the bad fats, sugar, and salt that lead to heart disease. Eliminating processed foods can have almost immediate effects on blood pressure; a plant-based diet can lower it by up to 30% in weeks. Because a plant-based diet naturally leads to weight loss, it causes the heart to work less hard but more efficiently, thereby also lowering blood pressure.

Other Benefits

People who eat a plant-based diet have significantly lower rates of obesity; in fact, the plant-based miracle diet is the single most effective way of losing weight and keeping it off. As previously mentioned, obesity is linked to many health problems, including heart and cardiovascular disease, type 2 diabetes, metabolic syndrome, and high levels of stress. While in the 20th century and earlier most disease was due to starvation and malnourishment, obesity-related diseases are actually the product of a combination of overnutrition (too many calories) and malnutrition (not enough vitamins, minerals, and fiber).

When fiber intake is increased and the body is getting (and absorbing) enough nutrients, the excess weight begins to melt off. With reduced levels of sugar, hormones such as insulin become stabilized. Hormonal diseases, such as metabolic syndrome, insulin resistance, and type 2 diabetes, start to reverse. The wall of the gut begins to heal itself and the microbiome becomes healthy, causing problems such as autoimmune diseases and IBS to disappear without any medicinal intervention. The mood elevates, alleviating or even eliminating psychological problems such as depression and anxiety. Hardened arterial walls begin to soften, causing blood pressure to lower and thereby reducing the risk of stroke and other heart diseases. Without trans fats and bad cholesterol, arterial blockages are reduced and even eliminated, allowing for blood to flow freely throughout the body.

In summary, the benefits of the plant-based diet simply cannot be overstated. One of its most immediate effects is that high levels of blood sugar and high blood pressure begin to drop and reach safe, stable levels. In addition, it allows the body to heal itself so that other diseases and health problems, such as high cholesterol, obesity, and autoimmune diseases, are able to resolve themselves.

Chapter 10:

Other Options and Diet

The Atkins Diet

The Atkins Diet took the United States by storm in the late 1990s and early 2000s. Dr. Robert C. Atkins promoted the diet and wrote a book about it in 1972. The theory behind it is that carbs are the reason we gain weight, so limiting carbs as much as possible leads to weight loss. People on the diet are advised to restrict consumption of any starchy or sugary foods, such as potatoes, bananas, wheat, apples, juice, and candy. The payoff is that they can eat as much protein (meat) and good fat as they want.

When Dr. Atkins began advocating this approach in the second half of the twentieth century, nutritionists and doctors were aghast. Fat was believed to be the enemy, and sugar was, for the most part, harmless (sugary processed foods like Snack Wells became popular during the 1980s and 1990s as diet foods). However, our understanding of nutrition has changed; we now understand that sugar is far worse, and fat in natural forms, such as olive oil and the fat in avocados, can actually be beneficial. Artificial fats, such as hydrogenated oils and trans fats, are to be avoided. Many people have boasted of being able to successfully lose weight on the Atkins diet. Proponents claim that it increases energy levels and actually reduces the risk of heart disease.

Unfortunately, the Atkins diet does not advocate exercise, claiming that it is not necessary for weight loss. Furthermore, the severely reduced consumption of carbs actually leads to eating fewer vegetables and almost no fruits, causing your body to not get the nutrients that it needs. Atkins is actually an animal-based diet.

The South Beach Diet

As the Atkins diet craze began to subside, the new South Beach diet began to rise in popularity. Its appeal over the Atkins diet was that it allowed for carbs to be incorporated. The push of the South Beach diet is the glycemic index, which determines whether particular carbs are good or bad. The glycemic index is a measure of how much and how quickly particular carbs will raise your blood sugar; whole grains are encouraged because they have a low glycemic index, while refined carbs and sugar are restricted because they have a high glycemic index. The South Beach diet promotes consumption of lean protein, whole grains, good fats, and fruits and vegetables.

One benefit of the South Beach diet is that it is more sustainable than the Atkins diet. The sheer amount of meat consumed on the Atkins diet is so high that on a global level, it is not environmentally sustainable. On a personal level, it can become very expensive, very quickly. Because the South Beach diet advocates a moderate intake of low-fat meat, such as chicken and fish, it is more environmentally and personally feasible. More people are able to follow it long-term because it allows for a moderate consumption of carbs. The higher intake of fruits and vegetables, over the Atkins diet, means that people on the South Beach diet are getting more nutrients. However, as you have previously read, the consumption of whole grains means more lectins, which lead to leaky gut syndrome.

The Paleo Diet

One of the latest diets to hit the US is the so-called paleo diet. The premise of the paleo diet is that our bodies evolved to process certain foods, the ones that our paleolithic ancestors ate. These foods included fruits and vegetables, lean meats, nuts and seeds, and fish. Modern farming began approximately 10,000 years ago; foods associated with modern farming are not compatible with the way that our bodies evolved. These foods include dairy, grains, and legumes. Modern processed foods and any added sugar are absolutely avoided.

The paleo diet has proven to be more beneficial than the Atkins or South Beach diets. Benefits of the paleo diet include decreased leptins, especially since grains and legumes are eliminated. It naturally includes a higher amount of fruits and vegetables to compensate for the lack of grains. Because our paleolithic ancestors were always active, the paleo diet advocates exercise every day; exercise has proven to be beneficial to both physical and emotional health. Even though the paleo diet is not a weight-loss formula, advocates say that they lose weight on it. They also have increased glucose tolerance, lower levels of triglycerides, and a stabilized appetite. However, the paleo diet does not address the problem of lectins.

Why the Plant-Based Diet is Best

The plant-based diet is the best of all of these other diet plans because, rather than being primarily a means to lose weight, it addresses the root causes of disease and advocates a healthy lifestyle. Reducing consumption of meat is shown to reduce blood pressure; eliminating it completely reduces it even more. In addition, raising animals for meat consumes far more environmental resources than growing the plants that underlie the plant-based diet. The plant-based diet addresses critical areas, such as the microbiome and lining of the intestines, that are ignored by even the paleo diet. The plant-based diet is better for humans and for the environment.

In summary, the plant-based diet is not a fad or a means for quick weight loss. While weight loss is a result, that is merely a side benefit. Its goal is overall health and well-being. In addition to being better for your own personal health, the plant-based diet is better for the environment.

Chapter 11:

Myths and Dangers

The world of health food and diets has become so commercialized that any diet comes with a host of critics and advocates, and along with them, seemingly contradictory information. If you do a Google search for veganism, vegetarianism, Atkins diet, plant-based diet, lectins, or any number of terms associated with healthy eating, you will receive so many different accounts, based on different information, that you may be tempted to forego healthy eating altogether. Knowing what to feed our bodies for optimal health and well-being seems to be the insurmountable task. There are some myths associated with the plant-based miracle diet, which this chapter will explain and dispel. It will also highlight some of the dangers of a plant-based diet, with the purpose of giving you the information you need to overcome them.

Myth 1: Whole grains and dairy are important sources of vital nutrients.

Despite the growing prevalence of leaky gut syndrome and increasing evidence that it is correlated with, if not caused by, dairy and the lectins found in whole grains, many nutritionists insist that both are necessary components of a healthy diet because of the nutrients found in them. However, there are no nutrients found in whole grains and dairy that can't be found elsewhere. Green, leafy vegetables, such as broccoli, kale, spinach, and parsley, are high in the B vitamins commonly found in whole grains but without the high level of lectins, as well as the calcium touted by dairy. Consuming these foods will not only reduce the amount of lectin you ingest and therefore help heal your intestinal lining but will also increase the prebiotics that feed your gut's microbiome.

Myth 2: Animal protein is superior to plant protein.

Other primates, including gorillas, have muscles that are far bigger than ours. However, they derive virtually all of their protein from plant sources. The fact is that amino acids are created by plants, which are then consumed by animals. Animals create some amino acids, but these can be obtained from plants. In fact, all plants contain all nine essential amino acids; therefore, consuming a sufficient amount of plant-based food will ensure that you get enough protein. The rule of thumb is that if you are getting enough calories from a plant-based diet, then you are getting enough protein.

Myth 3: A plant-based diet is prohibitively expensive.

Healthier food is certainly more expensive, especially when placed side-by-side with its processed counterparts. If a loaf of white bread costs one dollar and a loaf of sprouted-grain bread costs five dollars, one can easily conclude that healthy food is five times more expensive. However, that is only part of the actual situation.

Most Americans go out to eat between three and five times per week. If the average cost of a restaurant meal is ten dollars, then that is as much as fifty dollars a week going to unhealthy restaurant food! If you put that much money towards buying plant-based food rather than convenient restaurant food, you will probably end up spending about the same amount.

Many people on a plant-based diet report that they actually spend less on food than they previously did when eating a diet high in animal products and grains. Furthermore, they spend less on health-related issues, making the savings even more.

Myth 4: B12 is only found in meat.

Vitamin B12 is actually created by bacteria, not by animals. Animal products contain B12 because the bacteria in the animals create the B12. Properly fermented vegetable-based foods, such as natto (fermented soy), can be used to meet a person's B12 needs.

Danger 1: Plants don't contain Vitamin A in the form that our bodies need.

Our bodies need Vitamin A in the form of retinol, but what plants give us is beta-carotene, which is then converted into retinol. Based on conditions such as the health of your gut, your thyroid function, and some genetic factors, your body's ability to convert beta-carotene into retinol could be compromised. In order to avoid this danger, take the necessary steps to ensure that your gut is properly functioning so that it can properly convert beta-carotene into retinol. You may want to get a periodic blood test to ensure that you have appropriate levels of Vitamin A.

Danger 2: Not consuming animal products can reduce the amount of stomach acid, thereby reducing the overall efficiency of the digestive system.

When you consume animal products, especially meat, your stomach creates more hydrochloric acid (stomach acid) to assist in the breakdown of proteins. The digestive process is driven largely by a balanced pH, meaning that stomach acid is necessary to kick-start digestion. Without adequate stomach acid, the body is actually less able to absorb the nutrients that you consume. This condition is called hypochlorhydria. It results in abdominal discomfort, bloating, and gas immediately after eating and can lead to malnutrition from lack of nutrient absorption.

In order to prevent hypochlorhydria, drink a cup of room-temperature water with a tablespoon of apple cider vinegar before meals. The apple cider vinegar will help stimulate the stomach to produce the necessary acid.

Also, keep in mind that digestion is not merely a physical process. It is actually a parasympathetic process that involves both the mind and the body. Emotional distress can actually impede digestion. Maintaining a stress-free lifestyle and being relaxed when you eat can also combat hypochlorhydria.

In summary, many of the reasons why people decide not to follow the plant-based diet are based on faulty logic and science. There are no nutrients found in animal sources that cannot also be derived from plants, and usually with higher quality. While there are potential dangers in following the plant-based diet, they can be alleviated by taking simple measures.

CHAPTER 12:

THE IMPORTANCE OF NUTRITION

Even though Dr. Atkins claimed that exercise is not necessary for weight loss, it is a necessary aspect of overall health and well-being. Eighty percent of wellness is based on diet, while the other twenty percent is based on exercise. This chapter will look at that concept in more detail.

Eighty Percent Diet

It goes without saying that the food you eat is incredibly important. Proper nutrition can prevent many of the diseases associated with modern society and reverse them in people who already have them. This section will look at some important vitamins and minerals and give you information on what they do and what plant-based foods contain them.

Iron is a mineral usually obtained from red meat, but it is also present in green leafy vegetables, such as kale, spinach, and broccoli, as well as eggs and shellfish. It is required by red blood cells in order for them to transport oxygen throughout the body. Iron deficiency is known as anemia; it causes cells throughout the body to become hypoxic (lacking in oxygen). As a result, someone with anemia will feel weak, fatigued, and may even faint.

Vitamin D has gained a lot of popularity in the health community over the past few years, and for good reason. Its functions include allowing the body to absorb calcium, which is necessary for bone health, regulating the immune system so that it functions properly, and protecting against cancer. Low levels of vitamin D are linked with many different cancers, weight gain, heart disease, and depression. It can be obtained from egg yolks and wild fish, but the body actually produces it naturally from sunlight. In order to have optimum levels of vitamin D, the best thing to do is get plenty of sunshine.

Vitamin K is an unsung hero, as vitamin D has attracted so much attention. Vitamin K allows the blood to clot and aids in the transportation of calcium throughout the body, making it essential for healing injuries and protecting bone health. Without vitamin K, a simple wound can lead to so much blood flow that the injured person can resemble a hemophiliac. This important nutrient can be found in pretty much any fruit or vegetable that is green: Brussels sprouts, spinach, kiwi, avocado, broccoli, cabbage, kale, chard, and grapes.

Vitamin B1, or thiamine, is required by the body in order to process carbohydrates and proteins. Many people rely on whole grains to obtain thiamine, but it can also be found in nuts and some vegetables, such as peas.

Vitamin B2, or riboflavin, aids in the production of red blood cells and converting food into energy. Without an adequate supply of B2, no matter how many calories you consume, you will still feel lethargic. It can be obtained by eating almonds and asparagus and is also found in dark chicken meat.

Vitamin B6 is crucial because, like B2, it helps convert food into energy; it also aids in the breakdown of sugar, making it particularly beneficial for people who have developed insulin resistance or type 2 diabetes. It can be found in peas, spinach, and bananas; those who choose to consume small amounts of animal products can also find it in light poultry meat and eggs.

Vitamin C is touted for its ability to help boost people's immune systems. More than that, it is critical for the formation of collagen (the main protein found in the connective tissue between cells) and in creating some of the chemical messengers that the brain uses to transport its electrical signals. Sugary processed foods, such as gummy fruit snacks, and sugary juices like to boast of containing high levels of vitamin C; however, more than ample amounts of it can be found in nearly any fruit. Instead of drinking a glass of orange juice to help fight off a cold, eat a whole orange. You will get plenty of vitamin C that has not been subjected to the processing required to make orange juice; the whole orange will also provide you with the fiber needed to prevent a spike in blood sugar.

Vitamin E is a powerful antioxidant that protects cells from damage that can be incurred from toxins and the normal aging process. It is also important for skin health; medical professionals may apply pure vitamin E directly to a severe skin injury. It can be found in plant-based foods that are high in fat, such as olive oil, avocados, and nuts.

Keep in mind that while some oils, such as corn, soy, canola, and vegetable oil, are also derived from plants, they are created in laboratories and are full of damaging trans fats. They should be avoided as often as possible.

Folate is particularly important for pregnant women because it helps prevent birth defects. It also aids in heart health and in the creation of red blood cells. Many people rely on grains, beans, and lentils to obtain it, but it can be found in plentiful supply in dark green vegetables.

Calcium is important for healthy bone growth and development, as well as for transporting messages between cells and helping muscles work. Its benefits are widely touted as part of a campaign to get Americans to drink more milk; however, milk contributes to leaky gut syndrome. Furthermore, the calcium found in milk is not the best kind. The best calcium can be found in broccoli and dark leafy vegetables. For those who opt to consume animal products, it is also found in fish and fish bones (which are edible).

Magnesium is another unsung hero in the arsenal of vitamins and minerals. It improves nerve function, decreases anxiety, improves sleep, alleviates muscle pain, improves heart health, prevents migraines, and relieves constipation. This vital mineral can be found in dark leafy greens, nuts, avocados, and bananas. It can also be obtained by taking a bath with Epsom salt.

Zinc helps boost immune function so that you can heal faster. It strengthens the hair, skin, and nails, and a plentiful supply of zinc can even diminish scars! Many Americans obtain zinc through red meat and poultry, but it can also be found in nuts and seafood. Zinc supplements can also be beneficial but are no substitute for a good diet.

Twenty Percent Exercise

If twenty percent of health and well-being is dependent on exercise, then without it, even the most nutritious diet in the world will only bring eighty percent of your health potential. The twenty-percent deficit could leave you prone to depression, anxiety, and physiological disease. This section will look at different types of exercise and the benefits that they can produce.

Cardio exercise is basically any exercise that raises the heart rate. It includes brisk walking, running, swimming, stair stepping, bike riding, rowing, and dancing, amongst other things. Cardio exercise produces many benefits, beginning with promoting heart health. Muscles are healthier when they are used, and the heart is no exception. Elevating the heart rate during 30-minute to hour-and-a-half sessions of cardio workouts can strengthen the heart so that it actually creates more capillaries, thereby allowing blood to flow more freely throughout the body. It also burns off unwelcome substances that can build up in the blood and other parts of the body, such as triglycerides, excess sugar, and stress hormones. As a result, it leads to weight loss, increased energy, elevated mood, and decreased stress. Whatever your exercise routine may be, you should make time for at least thirty minutes of cardio most days of the week.

Strength exercises help to keep your bones and muscles strong. They include lifting weights and resistance training, such as using resistance bands or resistance machines. Strength exercise is not just for the young; older people in particular benefit from it because it helps them maintain their independence and prevent falls.

Flexibility exercises help maintain a wide range of motion while keeping your body limber. The range of motion refers to the extent to which you are able to move different parts of your body; people with conditions such as bursitis can benefit from flexibility exercises, as they can help extend the range of motion and thereby help the person get back his or her abilities. Flexibility exercises include doing yoga and stretching various parts of the body.

Balance exercises, such as tai chi, standing on one foot, some yoga positions, and heel-to-toe walking, help to strengthen the body's core. A stronger core promotes overall health, especially digestive and gut health, and decreases the risk of diseases that begin in the abdomen (such as type 2 diabetes and some autoimmune diseases).

In summary, the plant-based diet is able to provide you with all of the nutrients necessary to achieve optimal functioning of the entire body. Even nutrients typically obtained from meat, such as iron.

Chapter 13:

Safety, Side Effects, and Warnings

Despite its superior benefits, the plant-based miracle diet does not come without some of its vices. These vices, however, do not outweigh the benefits of the diet.

Many Americans are incredibly deficient in fiber; while 97% of Americans get enough protein (because of all the meat that they consume), 97% of Americans do not get enough fiber. The average fiber intake is only fifteen grams per day, while the body needs 32 grams per day! Switching to a plant-based diet means a significantly higher intake of fiber, which may take some adjusting. Common side effects of increased fiber intake include bloating, abdominal cramps, gas, and diarrhea. Less common side effects include temporary weight gain (usually from water) and constipation. In order to mitigate these side effects, make the switch to the plant-based diet gradually. Instead of immediately jumping from one or two servings of fruits and vegetables per day to ten, build that number up over the course of a few weeks. Not only will this allow your system to adjust, but it will also give you time to adjust your lifestyle to accommodate the plant-based diet.

One benefit of the plant-based diet is that it cleanses toxins that have accumulated in your body from years of unhealthy eating. Some people immediately feel great. However, for some people, this purge can lead to symptoms of detox, including aches and pains, fatigue, irritability, and other ailments commonly associated with the flu. Most Americans are addicted to sugar; sugar has actually hijacked their brains similar to narcotics and other addictive substances so that the brain is tricked into thinking that it has to have it. Switching to the plant-based diet may involve a withdrawal process, which can include anxiety, depression, intense cravings, moodiness, and brain fog. In order to mitigate these side effects, eat fruit whenever a sugar craving hits. Drinking a calming beverage, such as lemon balm tea, throughout the day can help lessen the anxiety and moodiness.

Consider the transition process, in which your body adjusts to the plant-based diet, as any transition process. Transitions are not ever easy. Think of it like getting a new puppy. The new puppy is cute, playful, and cuddly, so much so that you would not dream of getting rid of it. However, that puppy has to be house trained so as to not constantly do its business on the floor (or any other unwelcome place). This process involves completely changing your routine so that you are available every few hours to take the puppy outside. Furthermore, the puppy wants to chew on everything, including your expensive shoes. You have to learn to put all of your things away so that the puppy cannot chew on them, and will still have to replace some things that were important. However, as your routine adjusts to life with a puppy, you grow fond of it as it contributes to increasing your own happiness and quality of life. You love playing with it, and seeing it happy makes you happy. One day, you will look back on those days of adjustment to life with a puppy with fondness and won't even think about all the potty accidents or chewed-up shoes.

Likewise, when you make the transition to a plant-based diet, the process may be hard and require some serious adjusting. However, once your body gets used to it, you will feel so good and will have such an increased quality of life that you won't have any desire to go back.

Some people wonder whether the plant-based diet is for them. Simply put, the plant-based diet is for everyone. People of all ages and at all stages of life can benefit from it. Pregnant women who plan their meals appropriately can benefit immensely from the plant-based diet. It can counteract some of the fatigue and morning sickness brought on by pregnancy while still providing the developing baby with all of the nutrients necessary to thrive. In addition, pregnant women on the plant-based diet have a markedly lower chance of developing gestational diabetes and other pregnancy complications.

Children, even infants, can benefit from the plant-based diet. While infants need high levels of fat, this can be obtained from the mother's breast milk. Following the World Health Organization guidelines of breastfeeding for two years will ensure that your child will get all of the fat needed throughout the infant and toddler years. Children raised on the plant-based diet have fewer behavioral problems, including ADD and ADHD.

Athletes and bodybuilders are notorious for consuming large quantities of meat and other animal products in order to fuel their muscles for intense training sessions. However, they can get all of the nutrients that they need on a plant-based diet, especially one that calls for eating free-range, grass-fed meat once or twice a week. All of the nutrients needed for cellular and muscular growth and repair can be found in plants; small amounts of meat and other animal products can work as a supplement.

In summary, there are some drawbacks to the plant-based diet, but nothing that cannot be overcome. The uncomfortable effects of a drastic increase in fiber intake can be mitigated by gradually increasing the amount of fiber in the diet until optimal levels are achieved. The symptoms of detox that come from flushing the toxins from the body can be very uncomfortable, but again, a gradual transition can ease this process. Withdrawal from sugar addiction can be the hardest part of the transition for some people; to help get through it, eat a lot of fruit and drink herbal tea.

Chapter 14: The Light Dieters

Light dieters are individuals who want the benefits of the plant-based diet but are unable to make a commitment for a total change. They change one meal a day and aim to make the other two meals as healthy as possible. This chapter is specifically for people whose lifestyles may be inflexible due to occupational, financial, or any other reasons. Construction workers, athletes, shift workers, and others who need a lot of energy and are not able to take the time to deal with the side effects of going entirely plant-based are ideal candidates. People who want to experiment with the plant-based diet to see if it is something they can stick with are also ideal candidates. This regimen also applies to people who want to change to eating entirely a plant-based diet but are making the change gradually.

Changing One Meal a Day

Changing one meal a day from being meat-based to being plant-based is one way to substantially benefit your own health as well as the health of the planet. If every American switched one meal a week from being meat-based to being entirely vegan, the environmental equivalent would be like taking half a million cars off the road! To further increase the benefit both to your own health, the local economy, and the global environment make that one meal per day locally sourced from small farmers in your area.

The immediate benefits of changing one meal a day to being plant-based include that your daily servings of fruits and vegetables will go up. Many people rely on meat for their protein intake; however, some fruits and vegetables, such as jackfruit, are also high in protein as well as other vital vitamins and minerals. Choosing to use these plant-based sources of protein, even only one time each day, will provide the added benefit of extra fiber and other essential nutrients.

Your palate will expand as you try new fruits and vegetables that you previously had not even heard of. You may find that there are a lot of plant-based foods out there that you enjoy more than you did processed foods! This will encourage you to further increase your intake of a variety of fruits and vegetables and completely eliminate all processed foods. You may not even be tempted to go back to your old ways of eating.

Changing just one meal a day will allow you to gain many of the benefits of the plant-based diet, including improved overall health and vitality; reduction, reversal, and even elimination of chronic as well as acute diseases; and more energy. Furthermore, some of the unpleasant side effects — such as gas, bloating, diarrhea, and constipation — will be alleviated compared to those who make the full switch immediately. In other words, by changing just one meal a day to being completely plant-based, you should expect to feel better!

There is an important caveat, one known as the law of compensatory consumption. When we make positive changes, we tend to subconsciously justify doing more of our negative, detrimental habits because we feel so good about ourselves. For example, when people decide to use less water to help reduce their environmental footprints, they oftentimes subconsciously use more energy than they did previously; this is because they feel that their decreased water consumption justifies an increased use of electricity. People who switch to one plant-based meal a day will feel the temptation to eat more meat and processed foods at other meals. Be aware of this temptation so that you can resist it! Keep at the forefront of your mind the reason why you are making the switch to one plant-based meal per day so that you don't even want to eat more meat or processed foods. Don't fall prey to the law of compensatory consumption!

In summary, making the switch to eating one plant-based meal per day is a great way to kick off a lifestyle of healthy eating. You can begin to reap the benefits of the plant-based miracle diet but without many of the unpleasant side effects that can come with it. In addition, by making the change gradually, you are more likely to stick with the diet rather than if you jumped in all the way without giving yourself a transition period.

Chapter 15: Intermediate Dieters

Intermediate dieters are people who change two meals per day from being meat-based to being plant-based. Maybe they have already gone through the transition of changing one meal a day and can't get enough of the positive benefits. They want to continue making the switch to being entirely plant-based eaters. Other people who are ideal candidates for being intermediate dieters are those who have active social lives that include eating out with friends and/or family on a frequent basis. While restaurant meals almost inevitably contain animal products unless the menu says otherwise, eating a plant-based diet for two meals a day can compensate for the restaurant meals. In addition, busy moms whose families are resistant to eating a plant-based diet are ideal for changing two meals per day; they can eat a plant-based breakfast and lunch and then enjoy the same supper as their families. Meanwhile, all of the people making the switch to changing two meals a day from being meat-based to being plant-based are reaping even more of the rewards of the plant-based miracle diet.

Benefits, Expectations, and Results

The benefits of changing two meals per day from being meat-based to being plant-based are substantial. Most energy consumption in the sector of agriculture and food production comes from meat; it actually takes up to five times more water and a hundred times more food to produce a pound of meat as opposed to a pound of vegetables. The first benefit is a significantly reduced environmental impact. If the two plant-based meals that you eat each day are sourced from local small farmers and are organic (many small farmers use organic growing techniques, even if their produce is not certified as organic), the environmental impact is reduced even further. The second benefit is even more energy. While changing one meal a day to a plant-based diet increases energy levels substantially, changing two meals a day increases them even more. By giving your body the proper vitamins and minerals, as opposed to just the calories, that it needs, it is able to use the calories that it has consumed as energy. With that increased energy, you will *want* to exercise; rather than being a chore, exercise will become an indispensable part of your daily routine. Reaping all of the benefits of exercise is reason enough to make the change! Another benefit is increased alertness and improved mood. Brain fog, irritability, depression, and anxiety can all be caused, at least to an extent, by a poor diet that is high in processed foods and animal products. Eliminating processed foods and significantly reducing the number of animal products consumed can quickly turn those conditions around without any medication.

Just like with the one-meal-per-day switch, if you make the two-meal-per-day switch, you should expect to feel better. Your body will cleanse out more of the toxins that accumulated due to years of poor diet. While at first, you may experience some fatigue and withdrawal, especially if you didn't first make the transition to one plant-based meal per day, those effects are the result of your body being purged of all those toxins. After a few days, once your body has been cleansed, you will feel drastically better. Inflammation, and all of the problems that come with it — such as chronic aches and pains — will go down. Your gut will begin to heal, and its microbiome will be restored to optimal levels. In addition, excess weight will begin to fall off.

As with making the switch to one plant-based meal per day, make sure that you don't succumb to the law of compensatory consumption. Don't eat extra junk food to make up for all of the healthy food that you are now eating. If you must, splurge in another area. Get yourself a nice haircut or buy a new outfit to complement your now-healthy body. But don't steer off course! Then again, why would you even want to?

In summary, making the switch to eating two plant-based meals per day augments the benefits of eating one plant-based meal per day. Energy, vitality, and overall health and well-being are increased. The body flushes out the toxins that have accumulated and begins to heal itself, without the need for medication. The result is a happier and healthier you!

Chapter 16: Hard-Core Dieters

Hard-core dieting, in reference to the plant-based diet, is not an exercise in restriction or deprivation. Rather, it is a lifestyle of eating exclusively plant-based foods and reaping the benefits. While changing one or two meals a day is an ideal way for a lot of people to regain their health, especially people who are unwilling or unable to commit to an exclusively plant-based diet, going entirely vegan is for those who are completely committed to their health and well-being.

There are many lifestyle changes involved in eating nothing but the plant-based miracle diet. One of them is that socializing with friends will no longer involve going out to eat at any restaurant you or your friends should choose. Either the restaurant will have to have vegan options, or you will have to content yourself with watching everybody else eat. An alternative will be to invite friends over to your house for a vegan meal before going out on the town (or whatever you enjoy doing with your friends). An even better alternative is to not go solo when switching to the plant-based diet. See if any of your friends or family want to join in your endeavors. If no one wants to, at least try to earn the support of the people closest to you. That way, when you speak up about wanting to go to a restaurant that has vegan options, the people around you are more likely to acquiesce. They may even want to try vegan options, too!

Other lifestyle changes that you will probably encounter in the transition to full veganism include having to read food labels to determine if something is truly vegan and incorporating plant-based protein sources that aren't high in damaging lectins, such as natto. You will probably face some challenges in the transition, including the side effects mentioned in an earlier chapter. However, the benefits are life-changing.

People who went completely vegan for a mere 60 days reported that no matter how much they ate, they still lost weight. They experienced less soreness and had so much energy that they didn't know what to do with themselves. Six weeks in, they were prepared to make the transition permanent.

In summary, making the change to complete veganism is hard. It involves a lot of lifestyle changes and learning to eat in an entirely different way. However, it also leads to a revitalized body with exceptionally high energy levels.

CHAPTER 17: GOING ORGANIC

Dangers of Pesticide Use and Conventional Farming

In the year 1962, an American writer named Rachel Carson published a book entitled *Silent Spring*. The book highlighted how the use of heavy pesticides, including the supposedly safe one known as DDT, which was used commercially for agriculture and at home. The pesticide was known to cause cancer, yet was being sprayed indiscriminately into the environment. No long-term study had shown what its long-term environmental impact would be, but the bird population — including the emblematic bald eagle — was deteriorating because of its use. The title, *Silent Spring*, hearkened to the idea that with continued use of pesticides, we might experience a spring in which no birds sing. A public outcry ensued, which led to the banning of DDT in the year 1972.

Modern agricultural chemicals, however, may actually be worse than DDT. Glyphosate, the active ingredient in the commercially available pesticide Round-Up, was approved for use in 1974, shortly after the banning of DDT. Most bacteria are actually beneficial, especially those that comprise your gut's microbiome. Glyphosate actually kills most of the beneficial bacteria, both in the soil and in your gut. As a result, disease-causing bacteria are able to proliferate. It also damages the nutrients in the soil so that the plants are not able to properly absorb them, leading to sick plants and nutrient-deficient food. Glyphosate decreases the body's ability to detoxify foreign invaders and process organic compounds, further contributing to disease. Furthermore, it is toxic to human DNA, thereby holding the potential to devastate the entire human genome. It also disrupts the reproductive system, leading to problems such as infertility and birth defects.

Glyphosate has been linked with the rise of many diseases. For example, the rise in the use of glyphosate corresponds almost perfectly with the rise in autism spectrum disorder in children. It is a known carcinogen, meaning that it causes cancer, and may also be linked to Alzheimer's.

The environmental impact of glyphosate is unprecedented. It has built up in soils, damaging local micro-ecosystems. In fact, it has penetrated so deeply into the soil that it is contaminating water in the underground water table. Rainfall naturally causes glyphosate to runoff into streams and rivers, where it wreaks havoc on marine life. Fish are showing genetic abnormalities. Male fish are showing female characteristics, and some are even dying out. From rivers and streams, glyphosate makes its way into the ocean, where it continues its path of destruction. While Monsanto, the company that manufactures glyphosate, claims that it disintegrates rapidly, its residues can be detected in water two weeks to well over a month after exposure. In soil, it can be detected six months or longer after exposure.

Glyphosate is not even the worst chemical used commercially today. 2,4-D is the active ingredient herbicide found in many weed killers that can be bought at a store. Commercial farmers and local households use it to kill weeds. However, 2,4-D comprised about half of the chemical known as Agent Orange, which was sprayed indiscriminately in the jungles of Vietnam to help soldiers navigate them during the war. Agent Orange caused diseases in approximately one-quarter of the people exposed to it, including birth defects, genetic mutations, and cancer. The chemical that you may be using to spray your own yard to kill weeds may be one of the two ingredients that composed Agent Orange!

GMOs

In 1994, the Flavr Savr tomato, the first genetically modified food, was approved for commercial distribution and sale. Since then,

GMOs, or genetically modified organisms, have proliferated to such a degree that unless explicitly labeled otherwise, you can be almost certain that what you are eating was genetically modified. Not only are plants genetically modified, but some animals are, as well. In fact, the first documented case of successful genetic modification was a mouse, in 1973. Today, genetically modified salmon are sold at supermarkets across the country. Genetically modified fish, known as GloFish and adored for their vibrant colors, are sold as pets. Genetically modified mosquitoes have been released into the wild to combat malaria and other mosquito-borne diseases.

Genetic modification is usually done to create some purported benefit. For example, some bananas have been genetically modified to help increase the body's ability to process vitamin A, and other crops have been genetically modified to make them drought resistant. The process of genetic modification involves isolating a particular desired gene, such as one that enables a crop to survive with less water, and inserting it into the genome of the candidate plant's seeds. This artificial manipulation creates plants that actually don't exist in nature. In addition, the benefit that the GMO plant is supposed to bring just doesn't come. Supposedly drought-resistant GMO crops are not able to withstand water shortages; in fact, they tend to do poorer than their non-GMO counterparts.

Eighty percent of GMO crops around the world are genetically modified to be resistant to herbicides and pesticides, especially the dangerous pesticide glyphosate. In fact, the company that creates most GMO seeds, Monsanto, is the same company that produces Round-Up! Crops that are genetically modified to withstand high levels of glyphosate are termed "Roundup Ready," and are specifically cultivated to be sprayed with glyphosate. Estimates are that approximately 300 million pounds of Roundup are sprayed every year globally. With the known and documented effects of Roundup on both human and environmental health, one can only shudder at what its extensive use is doing. In response, the weeds that Round-Up is supposed to be killing, while preserving the crop plants, are actually developing resistance to the herbicide, meaning that higher and higher levels of it are required.

GMO food poses a double threat to humans. The first is that the altered DNA actually changes the DNA of the bacteria in the microbiome, making them unable to perform their functions, and even changes the DNA in some of your body's cells. It is actually disrupting the human genome! The second is that it is loaded with glyphosate, exposing you to higher and higher levels of this toxic chemical. That apple that you think is a healthy snack, unless labeled as being organic or non-GMO, could actually cause infertility, cancer, hormonal disruptions, and genetic mutations!

Benefits of Organic Farming Techniques

As opposed to conventional, large agriculture, which relies heavily on the use of agrichemicals and leads to problems such as soil degradation and wasted water, organic farming uses techniques that are beneficial to the environment. Instead of artificial fertilizers, organic farming uses natural fertilizers, such as manure and compost. Instead of dangerous chemicals, it uses pesticides that are naturally created by plants or even insects, such as ladybugs. To keep the soil fertile, crop rotation is used. Instead of working against the environment by using artificial means to grow crops, it works with the environment by utilizing natural forces to produce a chemical-free crop.

Benefits of Eating Organic Food

The benefits of eating organic food over conventionally grown food are tremendous. People who switch to organic food routinely find that problems such as food allergies completely disappear. This could be because modern farming techniques, especially the cultivation of genetically modified food, is creating food sensitivities and allergies in otherwise healthy people. Another benefit is that people who eat organic food have substantially lower levels of chemical residue in their bodies. Therefore, they experience fewer of the health problems associated with high herbicide and pesticide use. In addition, because chemical toxins are often stored in fat cells, reducing those toxins can actually allow you to lose weight without necessarily reducing calorie intake! Because organic food is grown in healthier soil that retains its nutrients, it can even have a higher nutrient content than its conventional counterpart. All in all, organic food is better for you and for the environment.

In summary, modern, conventional farming techniques are devastating the health of the human population and of the planet. Heavy chemical use is damaging entire ecosystems, and GMO foods are causing even more extensive damage. However, organic farming techniques and the consumption of organic food hold great potential for reversing both environmental and human health problems.

Chapter 18: Complement to a Healthier You

The Ketogenic Diet

Our long-ago ancestors did not eat three meals a day, like we do. They hunted and foraged for food, and if there was no food, they simply didn't eat. However, in most cases, they didn't starve. Rather, their bodies adapted to this lifestyle by burning off fat as a primary energy source rather than sugar. In modern society, sugar is the most-used energy source, so much so that traditional nutritional wisdom says that glucose (a type of sugar) is the body's primary energy source. This reinforces the false idea that we need to eat a lot of carbs. Our bodies are actually very capable of using fat as a primary energy source; in fact, from a metabolic perspective, fat is a more stable and sustainable form of energy than sugar.

Ketones are substances created by the liver when it breaks down fat, thereby creating energy. Ketones are also important for brain health and mental function, so getting the body to create more ketones improves both the mind and body. The diet actually was developed as a way of treating neurological disorders! Most of the time, our bodies primarily rely on glucose, a simple form of sugar derived from carbs, as energy. As a result, the fat that is stored in our bodies is not burned; therefore, we are unable to lose weight. The ketogenic diet is about significantly reducing the amount of carbs eaten so that the body begins to burn fat liver produces the ketones to generate energy. Starving the body of carbs forces it into a metabolic state known as ketosis, which literally means that ketones are being broken down.

On the ketogenic diet, carbs only account for five to ten percent of all calories consumed, and those carbs come exclusively from fruits and vegetables. Seventy-five percent of all calories come from fat, and the remaining ones come from protein. The high-fat content is crucial to establishing an optimal state of ketosis; a high-fat diet also decreases hunger and appetite, as well as cravings for carbs. The fats should come from healthy, natural sources, such as avocados, unprocessed cheese, nuts, eggs, and red meat. The protein is derived from these high-fat foods. Variations on the ketogenic diet include cycling, with five days on and two days of high-carb intake, higher protein intake (suitable for athletes and bodybuilders), and adding in carbs around your workout schedule.

Because the body's own fat stores are being used for energy, the ketogenic diet quickly leads to weight loss. In addition, it has many other benefits, as well. The extremely low intake of carbs leads to greater mental clarity and performance, leading to increased productivity. Without insulin being generated to aid in the transportation of glucose, people on the ketogenic diet become more energetic and have a more regulated sense of being hungry and full. Lower, stabilized insulin can reverse the effects of insulin resistance and even type 2 diabetes. People with acne tend to benefit from the ketogenic diet as well, as it helps lead to clearer skin. Despite the high amount of fats consumed, it actually lowers cholesterol and blood pressure. In addition, the ketogenic diet has been the primary method of treating children with epilepsy for over a hundred years. It reduces the amount of medication that they have to take and leads to better outcomes. The ketogenic diet is also believed to reduce the risk, symptoms, and progression of Alzheimer's disease and aid in recovery from brain trauma.

The ketogenic diet has been shown to improve insulin levels in people who are diabetic and prediabetic, thereby alleviating the symptoms and even the disease. However, people who are diabetic should only go on the ketogenic diet under a doctor's supervision.

Inability to create insulin means that glucose is unable to enter the cells to be used as energy, so the liver burns fats to create higher and higher levels of ketones. This can lead to a condition called ketoacidosis, which causes the body's pH to become so acidic that it can be fatal. Someone who does not have diabetes is at an immeasurably low risk of developing ketoacidosis; it usually only occurs in individuals whose diabetes is unmanaged.

Intermittent Fasting

Intermittent fasting is the process of starving the body of all calories so that it is forced into a metabolic state in which body fat is quickly burned and muscle is easily built. The idea behind it is that what you eat is not as important as when you eat; therefore, you don't have to give up any of the foods that you enjoy. Instead, you should only eat at certain times.

When food is consumed, the body spends about five hours digesting it; during digestion, hormones that lead to weight gain, especially insulin, are activated. Because most people eat within five hours of their last meal or snack, they are unable to enter into the stage in which they can lose weight because the fat-storing, weight-gaining hormones are constantly coursing through them. Intentionally foregoing meals by going through periods of fasting and feeding put the body into a state in which body fat is burned. You can drink as much water and calorie-free beverages (such as green tea and coffee) as you want but only eat at certain times. Fasting times usually range from 12 to 20 hours, but some programs have fasting periods that last as long as 36 hours.

The idea of intermittent fasting goes against traditional nutritional advice, which says that in order to keep the metabolism moving, you need to eat small meals all throughout the day. Eating small meals leads to a higher metabolic rate, while foregoing food puts the body into starvation mode, causing the metabolism to slow down and fat to be stockpiled. The problem with this traditional wisdom is that it is built on the idea that glucose, rather than fat, should be the body's primary energy source. In order for the body to continually provide energy through glucose, there does need to be a constant supply of food. However, that glucose raises insulin levels, leading to weight gain, not weight loss. The wisdom of intermittent fasting is that it relies on lowering insulin levels so that the body burns fat with little effort.

There are several different intermittent fasting programs,

including LeanGains, the Warrior Diet, Fat Loss Forever, the Alternate Day Diet, and Eat Stop Eat. The Warrior Diet was one of the first diets to bring in the idea of intermittent fasting. It is based on the concept that in ancient civilizations (and even sometimes in modern ones), warriors or soldiers did not stop during the day to eat. Rather, they marched, trained, and battled during the day and only ate in the evenings. However, they were fit, alert, and capable of facing the enemy. On the Warrior Diet, you fast for 20 hours every day and consume all of your daily nutritional needs within a four-hour feeding window in the evenings. This regimen can be difficult to adopt all at once, so people on the Warrior Diet usually transition into it gradually. LeanGains is an intermittent fasting plan that incorporates workouts into the fasting and feeding schedule so as to optimize fat burn and muscle build. Other intermittent fasting plans, such as Fat Loss Forever and the Alternate Day Diet, use various schedules of feeding, fasting, and workouts so as to get the best results.

The benefits of intermittent fasting go beyond weight loss; it also helps improve cardiovascular health, energy levels, and mental clarity. Adjusting to intermittent fasting can be challenging, especially because until the body fully adjusts, periods of fasting can involve intense hunger, irritability, anxiety, and moodiness. Given time, the body is usually able to adjust quite well so as to reap the benefits of intermittent fasting. Some religious groups already advocate intermittent fasting, such as Muslims who fast during Ramadan. If fasting is already a part of your spiritual life, then intermittent fasting can be a way to kill two birds with one stone; you can get both the physical and spiritual benefits.

Many people can benefit from intermittent fasting. Those who have been trying to lose those last five or ten pounds, people who enjoy working out frequently, and people who already fast for reasons other than weight loss can benefit from implementing an intermittent fasting regimen. Pregnant women and people with certain diseases, including diabetes and ones that require a ketogenic diet (as opposed to being on a ketogenic diet voluntarily), should not try intermittent fasting. Additionally, some people have difficult schedules that can make intermittent fasting difficult, if not impossible. College students, shift workers, and people who must be on-call for work may have a very difficult time adapting an intermittent fasting program into their lifestyles. They may want to try another health and wellness program, such as the plant-based miracle diet or the ketogenic diet.

For more information, you can check out my book on intermittent fasting.

Exercise

The benefits of exercise are well-known and documented. People who exercise regularly experience lower levels of disease, higher levels of energy, a more moderated appetite, and higher overall health and well-being. Many people have been able to get off of a variety of medicines, everything from antidepressants to statins, because exercise alone was enough to alleviate the symptoms and even cure the underlying cause of illness. In order to get the most out of exercise, you need to get your heart rate above normal. While adding casual walks into your daily routine is beneficial in many ways, vigorous exercise that gets the heart pumping and forces you to breathe harder is the best. A brisk morning walk, taking the stairs at work, and a trip to the gym are all great ways to add heart-healthy exercise into your daily regimen.

Accountability Partners

Accountability partners are an important component of staying on track as you make the lifestyle changes necessary to become healthier. Your accountability partner may be someone who is more of a mentor that has already gone through the process; this mentorship set-up has shown to have great results in programs like Alcoholics Anonymous. Your accountability partner may also be a friend or peer who, like you, wants to get healthy. People who have accountability partners are much more successful at reaching their overall goals.

The key to having an effective accountability partnership is easy: Stay accountable to each other! Plan to connect with each other at least once a week to share how that week has been going. Did you fall off the wagon and into the sugar trap? Did you have a meat craving that you just couldn't ignore? How does your accountability partner deal with cravings? What are some of the benefits that you are seeing from your lifestyle changes? An accountability partner can give you an extra layer of vision that you don't have on your own because he or she can see things that you cannot. For example, you may see that the numbers on the scale haven't budged, but your accountability partner may notice that you look slimmer and your skin is brighter. He or she can also give you tips on other lifestyle changes that you can work into your daily or weekly routine.

Staying Motivated

Staying motivated while on a healthy eating lifestyle can be challenging sometimes, especially when you hit a weight-loss plateau (in which you are no longer able to lose weight) or when the holidays come around. Having an accountability partner and focusing on all the benefits that you are already seeing from your healthy eating lifestyle can help you stay on track. But what about in the beginning, when your whole body is sore from the toxins being purged from it and you don't think you will survive another sugar craving?

One necessary component of staying motivated is to make one change at a time rather than jumping in headfirst. Each time you make a change, be sure to replace the original with something even better. That way, you are easing yourself into a positive transition in which you actually like the replacement better; the changes will be much longer lasting than if you focus on deprivation and what you can't have. First, focus on eliminating sugar from your diet. Are you a heavy soda drinker? Start there. Throw out all the soda and get rid of all the excuses for needing it. No, you don't need to raise your blood sugar with a soda and no, you don't need the caffeine in it. Find a sugar-free alternative (not diet soda or anything that contains artificial sweeteners!). Kombucha is a fermented tea that still has a fizzy, slightly sweet taste but, unlike soda, has health-boosting probiotics, vitamins, and minerals. Many people have found that kombucha is a great alternative to soda. While it can be expensive to purchase (one bottle usually costs around three dollars), you can learn to make it at home for pennies a gallon.

Once the soda habit is gone, move on to your next sugar vice. Is it ice cream? A mid-afternoon crash that you solve with something sweet? Donuts? Find a suitable replacement for those things; instead of ice cream, use frozen bananas to make a smooth and creamy frozen snack. Eat frozen grapes; they can be a great way to satisfy a sweet tooth. For the mid-afternoon crash, plan ahead with a fruit salad that you will eat instead of going to the vending machine. Not only will you satisfy the need for something sweet, but you will have given your body an infusion of vitamins and minerals.

After a while, the gradual changes will start to snowball into a major lifestyle overhaul. Without you even thinking about it, that one vegan meal a day will become two. You'll want to take the stairs instead of the elevator because you love the feeling of getting the blood flowing. Give yourself enough choices, and you won't even miss the things that you thought you couldn't live without.

Habit Formation

Habits take between two weeks and one month to form. During the time when a habit is being formed, one slip-up can derail the entire process. The trick to forming a habit is to be aware of that fact so that you are equipped to not let those inevitable slip-ups get you completely off-track. Maybe you planned to go to the gym every Tuesday, Thursday, and Saturday. This Saturday, though, you just couldn't bring yourself to do it. Instead, you watched Netflix and ate grilled cheese sandwiches and drank soda. Before the end of the first season that you are binging on, you have convinced yourself that this healthy-eating lifestyle isn't for you and you can't do it, anyway. All of the efforts that you put into creating the necessary habits to enforce your lifestyle changes could easily be derailed at that point unless you are already aware of that potential.

The good news is that everybody has slip-ups. Everybody has bad days. And the best news is that that's perfectly OK! So, you had pizza delivered and ate four slices while going through two seasons of Game of Thrones instead of going to the gym. That does not make you a failure. It just means that you need to get up and start again tomorrow. Be kind to yourself, let yourself have a bad day, and then get back on track.

One key to preventing those slip-ups from becoming a regular occurrence is to try to figure out what causes them. Are you an emotional eater? Maybe a particularly stressful event or just feeling overwhelmed, rather than your own lack of willpower, led to you downing a pint of ice cream. Keep a journal so that you can stay on track of what keeps you motivated (what enables you to stay strong on good days) and what leads to you having a splurge.

Thirty days of healthy eating and regular exercise is usually enough to enforce the new lifestyle. However, remember that the most long-lasting changes are those that come gradually, so if you aren't able to become an immediate vegan and stay on track for 30 days, it's probably because you're trying to do too much at once. Get off of sugar for 30 days, and you will find that you no longer even want sweets. Then get off all processed food for 30 days, and you will find that you only want food that is fresh and nutritious. Next, exercise regularly for 30 days. You will find that you want to do it every day! Congratulations. You just developed the necessary habits to stay on track.

Foods to Focus on

One key to staying on track is to keep your eyes on the foods that you can focus on; there are far more foods that you can eat to support a healthy diet and lifestyle than foods that can derail it. Focus on continually expanding your palate to include more of the great variety of natural, plant-based foods that can help lead to overall health and well-being. Focus on eating plant-based foods that are grown without agrichemicals, to ensure that those toxins don't end up inside your body.

Fiber is a nutrient that passes through the digestive system unaltered; however, it slows the absorption of sugar and keeps you feeling full longer. Foods that are high in fiber should be consumed consistently. This does not include processed foods that have fiber artificially added to them, like Metamucil crackers or fiber powder. Rather, it refers to foods that are naturally high in fiber. Vegetables that are particularly high in fiber include celery, carrots, artichokes, Brussels sprouts, and broccoli. Fruits that are high in fiber include berries (raspberries, blackberries, strawberries, and blueberries), avocados, apples, oranges, and pears. The best part about eating fiber-rich fruit is that even though it is sweet enough to satisfy a sugar craving, the fiber in it keeps your blood sugar and insulin levels from spiking. To ensure that the fiber isn't destroyed, try to eat fruits and vegetables uncooked as much as possible.

Other foods that should be focused on are foods that are bright and colorful. While sweet potatoes are technically starches rather than vegetables, they have a nutrient profile that can rival most vegetables, while having a sweetness that can make them even more satisfying than white potatoes. Spirulina and chlorella are algae that are loaded with B vitamins; they make a great addition to smoothies. Turmeric is a bright yellow-orange seasoning that has health benefits so strong that it is superior to many medications! Experiment by using as many natural herbs and seasonings in your cooking as you can.

Work on continually expanding your palate to include more colorful fruits and vegetables. When you are first trying new ones, start by adding them to smoothies, soups, or salads so that you can adjust to the taste. You will find that there are plenty of foods that your taste buds are just waiting to discover and enjoy!

Foods to Avoid

On any healthy-eating plan, the first group of foods that should absolutely be avoided is anything that causes a spike in insulin levels. High insulin levels are behind many cases of obesity and disease, so keeping your insulin stable is necessary to getting your health back.

Sugar, juice, white bread, soda, and pasta are just a few examples of insulin-spiking foods that should be avoided at all costs.

Lectins are substances found in plant proteins that can contribute to leaky gut syndrome, a condition in which the lining of the intestines becomes porous, allowing undigested food and toxins directly into the body. Virtually all foods contain lectins, so they cannot be completely avoided. However, some foods contain very high levels of lectins and should not be consumed. Beans and pulses, including kidney beans, navy beans, fava beans, lima beans, pinto beans, soybeans, mung beans, peas, and lentils are all high in lectins. Cooking destroys some of them, but not all. Grains and cereals, especially whole grains (because most of the lectins are found in the shell of the seed), are particularly high in lectins. These foods include barley, wheat, corn, rice, and wheat germ.

Genetically modified organisms (GMO food) should be avoided like the plague. Genetic modification alters the genome of an organism so that it is essentially a new breed that is not recognized in nature. The altered DNA can actually alter the DNA in your body's cells! In addition, GMOs are heavily sprayed with glyphosate, an herbicide that is known to cause cancer, hormonal disruptions, infertility, and a host of other health problems. In addition to the dangers GMOs pose to human health, they literally have the potential to completely destroy the planet. They inhibit biodiversity, which is crucial to healthy ecosystems. The glyphosate used to treat them has penetrated the water table, heavily contaminated the soil, and is wreaking havoc on marine and another animal life.

Supplements

Before considering taking supplements, remember that most of your nutritional needs should be met from the food that you eat. Supplements should be used only to enhance the nutritional benefits of food or to take the place of foods that you are unable to eat (for example, vegans often need to take supplements for the B complex). Use supplements in their most whole, natural form rather than chemically based supplements. For example, if you must use protein powder, use a brand that does not include chemicals in the powder and derives the protein from natural, rather than artificial, sources. Spirulina, chlorella, hemp, and chia seeds all make great supplements because they are entirely natural, come from plant-based sources, and can be added to food to make it more nutritious.

Some supplements can actually work adversely together to create a toxic brew in your blood. Talk to a doctor or pharmacist to ensure that any combination of supplements that you are taking is healthy.

Conclusion

Eating a plant-based diet is not a difficult one to follow IF you begin to look at food in the sense of vitamins and nutrients. The health benefits from becoming herbivorous, like having a clearer complexion, a healthier cardiovascular system, a reduced cancer risk, slow ever development of dementia symptoms, less painful joints, and feeling more energetic should be enough for anyone to make the switch. There are many studies that show plant-based diets to be one of the healthiest diets out there. This meal plan is 4 weeks of a basic plant-based plan. It will help keep you full and energized and will keep you from becoming deficient in necessary vitamins and nutrients.

If you become informed of where to get your entire daily nutrition, the transition into this diet should be a breeze; I have explained basic vitamins that people become easily deficient and where to get them. If you were unsure you would be getting all your nutrition from plants, never fear… plants have everything you need. Without eggs, dairy, or meat, you take away the countless problems that come which consuming these products. Unfortunately, the Earth must suffer as well. Because of all the livestock need to sustain the human population, there are more greenhouse emissions coming from the 60 billion livestock that are being emitted from all vehicles. That is extremely shocking; not only could we change our bodies, but we could also change the worl

www.ingramcontent.com/pod-product-compliance
Lightning Source LLC
LaVergne TN
LVHW010226070526
838199LV00062B/4729